EMPOWER A HEALTHIER YOU

DOING
DIABETES
DIFFERENTLY

CHAD T. LEWIS

Including a foreword by

DR. IRL HIRSCH & DR. STEPHEN PONDER

Commentaries by Riva Greenberg, Ginger Vieira,
Dr. Jody Stanislaw, Delaine Wright, and Dr. Randy Elde

RIVER GROVE
BOOKS

This book is intended as a reference volume only, not as a medical manual. The information given here is designed to help you make informed decisions about your health. It is not intended as a substitute for any treatment that may have been prescribed by your doctor. If you suspect that you have a medical problem, you should seek competent medical help. You should not begin a new health regimen without first consulting a medical professional.

Published by River Grove Books
Austin, TX
www.rivergrovebooks.com

Distributed by River Grove Books

Design and composition by Greenleaf Book Group
Cover design by Greenleaf Book Group

Publisher's Cataloging-in-Publication data is available.

Print ISBN: 978-1-63299-599-5

eBook ISBN: 978-1-63299-600-8

First Edition

To Drs. Laird Findlay, Irl Hirsch,
and Richard Bernstein, and Patty—
people who saved my life

CONTENTS

FOREWORD

Dr. Hirsch

When insulin was discovered one hundred years ago, it was thought by many to be a "miracle cure." Soon after, it was clear that wasn't the case. Fast-forward to the 1980s, and patients were told that, with the new insulin pumps and human insulin, they could eat whatever they wanted whenever they wanted. Again, sadly that wasn't the case at all.

While there are many diabetes books to read, few can give such a large amount of information and with so much detail as *Doing Diabetes Differently*. Warning: This is not a book to buy on the day you or a family member are diagnosed with diabetes. Many of the topics and concepts are more sophisticated, and in fact, you would think Chad is a certified health care professional with his knowledge. But Chad's credentials are unimportant.

The greatest strength of this book is the attention provided for lifestyle, perhaps the least discussed topic when visiting a physician for routine diabetes management. The reason for this is understandable: In medical school or primary care residency curricula, very little attention is provided for nutrition and exercise *as it pertains to diabetes management*. When reading this book, it will become clear that some of Chad's comments are controversial. *This is a good thing!* We will never have randomized controlled trials on each aspect of nutrition or exercise, and on how much of this can be related to items also important to overall health such as anxiety, guilt, depression, and yes, even finances.

Aims of any article or book include making the reader more knowledgeable in addition to providing a new way to think about challenges, in this case with diabetes management. The ultimate goal would be to cause behavior changes. Being newly diagnosed with diabetes or even starting a new medication for many does not result in changes in lifestyle. *Doing Diabetes Differently* challenges the reader to think more critically about what they've been taught or how they've been living their life with diabetes.

—Irl B. Hirsch, MD, Professor of Medicine,
University of Washington School of Medicine

Dr. Ponder

Taking charge of one's life and health is an aspirational goal of mature adults. *Doing Diabetes Differently* aims at empowering the busy adult seeking to balance a full life while maintaining effective control over the ever-capricious *diabetes mellitus*.

I first met Chad in San Diego at a national conference. Chad

had read my book *Sugar Surfing* and attended the presentation I delivered on it at the conference. Afterward, we had several in-depth existential exchanges about our diabetes and the paths we had both taken through life with it.

Chad and I quickly recognized the common bond we shared in regard to wishing to share what we had learned through our experiences. In my case, it originated from blending my half-century living with type 1 diabetes with three decades as a clinician and researcher in the field.

Chad's life experiences, combined with his deep intellect, academic accomplishments, and critical thinking skills, make him an ideal vehicle to challenge the status quo of current diabetes self-care paradigms. At the time, Chad shared with me that he was already planning a carefully researched and vetted book aimed at the busy adult with diabetes who is "looking for more" than a formulaic approach to self-care.

Chad approaches this focused book with a passion to share what he has learned. The book takes a refreshing approach that aims to challenge the reader's assumptions about diabetes care. He clearly separates the wheat from the chaff with style and grace and successfully achieves his objective of helping the reader to frame good questions of their care providers. Those of us involved with diabetes care will also benefit from the reading.

Chad's keen intellect and avoidance of common cognitive traps makes this an informative and insightful book. It's a must-read!

—Stephen W. Ponder, MD, FAAP, DCES, Professor, Joslin Medalist, and author of *Sugar Surfing: How to Manage Type 1 Diabetes in a Modern World*

INTRODUCTION

I write to all persons with diabetes.* Although the disease has many faces, those of us with the condition are more alike than different in the challenges we face.

Maybe you're new to the disease, or perhaps it's been part of your life for years. Either way, I assume you've picked up basic information and might be using medication to manage your blood sugar. But things aren't working out. Your average blood sugars are too high. You may be insulin-dependent and experiencing too many lows. You may be on a glycemic roller coaster.

---

* I could have written "diabetic" here. But using *diabetic* as a noun is viewed as being insensitive by some, and doing so was discontinued by the American Diabetes Association in 2016. (After all, we should be defined by *who* we are, as opposed to *what* we are.) I avoid the term or use it sparingly throughout the book, even though viewing oneself as being "a diabetic" can be helpful for reasons covered in Chapter 3.

Care providers may have added more layers of medication. You're knocking yourself out with prescriptions to lower blood sugar as you try to eat correctly.

You've found yourself insanely doing the same things repeatedly while expecting different, favorable results. You're frustrated, distressed, and seeking answers, and you feel the need to do diabetes differently. If that's the case, this book is for you.

Doing Diabetes Differently offers answers in the form of carefully researched frameworks and perspectives, many of which are not taught in medical school. This book shows the importance of the mental part of diabetes and covers an approach for managing it that goes beyond just treating the symptoms of diabetes distress. You'll learn the futility of "dieting" and the *what* and *why* of dietary alternatives that work. The book also offers a new perspective on exercise and a doable way to make it happen. You'll learn why less is more when it comes to diabetes drugs, including insulin, and how this can help your pocketbook. You'll see how all the parts of a diabetes life—related to mental demands, nutrition, exercise, and drugs and devices—fit together in a framework for healthy living.

The book doesn't offer up answers just from me. I realized that other voices were needed, including some that may not always agree with me. Accordingly, I invited diabetes experts to add commentaries that appear throughout the book. These experts and the foreword authors constitute a *Who's Who* in the US diabetes community: Dr. Randy Elde, Riva Greenberg, Dr. Irl Hirsch, Dr. Stephen Ponder, Dr. Jody Stanislaw, Ginger Vieira, and Delaine Wright.

Others who influenced the book's content include internist Dr. Laird Findlay; diabetes medical writer Carol Verderese; clinical nutritionist Karl Minicin; Children with Diabetes founder Jeff Hitchcock; diabetes author, educator, columnist, and blogger Wil Dubois; and Amber Clour, cofounder of the *Diabetes Daily Grind* and host of *Real Life Diabetes Podcast.*

Doing Diabetes Differently includes questions as well as answers. Each chapter concludes with questions you might ask your care providers—endocrinologist, primary care physician, diabetes care and education specialist (DCES), or nutritionist.[†] Other sense-making material includes recommended readings and other resources by topic. One-stop shopping! In this book, by topic, you'll discover a diabetes answer, a question you might ask to get one, or a reference you might consult to find one.

I promise that my writing goes well beyond a how-to manual based on a singular ray of light. I didn't write an "If I can do it, so can you!" trope. I also don't slam diabetes standard practice and conventional wisdom and, in the process, invent the One Best Way. Most definitely, I am *not* suggesting that you disregard your health care providers. On the contrary, my goal is to help you have more active and productive conversations with them. Occasionally, I do this by respectfully bouncing off established positions and published work of the American Diabetes Association (ADA) and various experts. But I don't grind an ax. We're all in this together.

A few words about why I wrote the book: Over the decades of living with type 1 diabetes, I've grown weary of watching people, especially my friends, being challenged by complications and even dying. Consequently, I decided to write a book to help people do the disease differently and better. I also wrote in the

---

† The terms "dietitian" and "nutritionist" are often used interchangeably. However, dietitians have higher education and certification standards, so I use the term "nutritionist" to capture the broader universe of all diet advisor professionals.

hope of expanding the conversation within the diabetes community, especially among care providers.

Also, I wrote to give back. Sales from *Doing Diabetes Differently* will benefit the Diabetes Daily Grind, a nonprofit organization dedicated to providing real support and resources for all people living with diabetes (diabetesdailygrind.com).

The views expressed herein are mine. Also, this is the place where I formally assert that I'm not a diabetes educator, nutritionist, exercise physiologist, or physician. I make no claims on which you should rely without active consultation with your health care providers. Indeed, a purpose of this book is to help you do this.

CHAPTER 1

THE SCOURGE

Diabetes doesn't often appear as a cause of death in obituaries or on death certificates. Of course, bereaved obituary writers may leave out such causes, or another cause is given: heart attack, stroke, kidney disease, and so forth.

The recent death of my friend Les was blamed on a heart attack rather than the real cause—diabetes. Les, a physically fit airborne Army Ranger during the Vietnam era, died in a hospital bed immobilized by diabetic vascular complications and neuropathy. Another friend, Jim, endured twelve hours of kidney dialysis each week and had a leg and the fingers on both hands amputated. He officially died from kidney failure, but diabetes was his real killer.

It's a daily struggle for the diabetic friends I still have with me. My weekly breakfast buddy at Wayne's Corner Cafe here on Camano Island, Washington, no longer goes crabbing; nor can he engage in other island adventures because of debilitating diabetic neuropathy. Another friend struggles, despite using the latest and greatest hybrid closed-loop insulin pump system.

I'm tired of my friends being taken down by a metabolic disorder. Hindsight is 20/20, but I believe their diabetes journey would have differed had they benefited from this book early on and done diabetes differently and better. The same may be true of you as well.

What Are We Talking About?

Making sense of diabetes begins with understanding what it is.

Diabetes is a metabolic disorder in which the body cannot properly use dietary macronutrients, especially carbohydrates. Carbs go beyond simple sugars found in foods like candy, pie, and cake. They include the complex carbohydrates found in supposedly healthy whole-grain bread, the fructose in fruit, and the lactose in milk. Even vegetables such as corn, carrots, and beets are full of carbs.

Eventually, except for some carbohydrates classified as dietary fiber, all carbs convert to circulating blood glucose. Dietary protein and fat also affect blood glucose (protein more so than fat). Circulating glucose signals beta cells in the pancreas to produce insulin that, in turn, lets glucose into body cells for energy, thereby stabilizing blood sugar levels at healthy, lower levels. Diabetes is diagnosed when blood sugar rises to unhealthy levels because beta cells are destroyed or can otherwise no longer do their job.

High blood sugars are associated with diabetic complications. High-glycemic variability (frequent highs and lows on the glycemic roller coaster) also contribute to complication risk.[1] In the United States, diabetes is the leading cause of blindness, impotence, and neuropathy (which can lead to amputations), and kidney disease (which often leads to dialysis and death). Across studies, people with diabetes are up to five times more likely to have a heart attack or stroke than are nondiabetics.

TYPE 2

Over 90 percent of those with diabetes have type 2 diabetes (T2D). Most experience metabolic syndrome, the label given to a physiological process that leads to both insulin resistance (a reduction in insulin's capability to transport glucose into cells for use as energy) and the eventual inefficiency or failure of insulin-producing beta cells in the pancreas. When people experience insulin resistance, they need more of it, so pancreatic beta cells respond by producing more insulin. Simultaneously, beta cells start to die or otherwise become dysfunctional, which overloads the surviving beta cells left behind. As average blood glucose rises precipitously, full-blown type 2 diabetes is diagnosed.

Metabolic syndrome is associated with several risk factors: excessive belly fat in apple- versus pear-shaped individuals, high blood sugars toxic to beta cells, a poor diet high in both fat and carbohydrates, a sedentary lifestyle, and genetics. The underlying physiology is complex. One study identifies *eight* different pathophysiological mechanisms involving insulin resistance and beta cell function that occur in insolation, or combination, that can lead to type 2 diabetes.[2]

Type 2 diabetes and being overweight go hand in hand. The condition is even referred to as "diabesity" in the literature.[3] Over 85 percent of those with T2D are overweight or obese; even being slightly overweight increases the risk of diabetes by five times. But being significantly obese increases the chances of type 2 diabetes by *sixty times*.[4] Height-weight-proportionate people with T2D are a puzzle, though. Nephrologist Jason Fung still attributes this, along with genetics, to excessive fat that's less visible because it is visceral as opposed to abdominal.[5]

Obesity is defined in the United States as having a body mass index (BMI) of 30 or greater. A BMI of 25 to 30 is simply overweight. A 5'11" man is obese at 215 pounds; a 5'2" woman, at 145. The *average* American comes close to these numbers. Based on the Centers for Disease Control and Prevention (CDC) data, the average American man is 5'9" and weighs 198 pounds; the average woman is 5'4" and weighs 171 pounds.[6] Go to any retail store or shopping mall in the United States and look around. A 5'9" male shopper weighing in at 198 pounds looks normal relative to everyone else walking by. Television programs have jumped on the bandwagon, with titles such as *My 600 Lb. Life*, *Family by the Ton*, *1000-Lb Sisters*, and *The Biggest Loser*. "Fat shaming" is discouraged in society, and that's a good thing. However, as individuals, should we also accept being overweight or obese as okay because it's commonplace?

T2D usually surfaces later in life. After years of poor nutrition, little exercise, and a growing waistband, a person with T2D might go to the doctor because of a funny numbness in their feet, or a man might have become impotent. There might be vision problems. Whatever the complaint, T2D is diagnosed, and diabetes education typically follows.

A person with T2D is usually told they can live a long and normal life *if* they lose weight, exercise, *and* eat a balanced, healthy diet. Sometimes metformin, a drug that slows down the release of glycogen (stored sugar) in the liver and muscles, is also prescribed. But things often don't work out. The person keeps gaining weight and blood sugar remains high, so another drug or two (possibly a DPP-4 inhibitor, a GLP-1 agonist, an SGLT-2 inhibitor, a TZD [thiazolidinedione], a sulfonylurea, or a megli-tinide) is added to the regimen to drive down hemoglobin A1c, a measure of blood sugar control over a two- to three-month period. A1c values may improve initially. Then, they don't.

All along, the health care provider may talk about the need for dieting and exercise and may even refer the T2D patient to a nutritionist, exercise physiologist, or both. But these interventions may still not work. The patient may be perceived to be uncooperative or "noncompliant." Eventually, as diabetes worsens, the prescribing care provider cuts to the chase and adds basal insulin to the mix. Eventually, mealtime boluses of fast-acting insulin may be added. All along, the drug regimen may include medication for the high blood pressure common in overweight or obese individuals and a statin to lower cholesterol. The person with type 2 diabetes might end up taking four, five, or more medications a day.

Again, A1c levels may improve until they don't. The person continues to battle weight gain. Complications progress. In the worst case, the person with type 2 diabetes falls apart and dies at a younger age than they might have, often from the cardiovascular disease that killed my friend Les or the kidney failure that killed my friend Jim.

TYPE 1

Type 1 diabetes, the other main type of diabetes, afflicts just 10 percent of the diabetic population. It occurs because of an autoimmune reaction that kills insulin-producing pancreatic islet cells. Myriad causes have been attributed to triggering this autoimmune reaction, such as drinking cow's milk as an infant, being exposed to a virus, and stress, to name a few, all accompanied by having a genetic predisposition.[7]

As insulin-producing pancreatic beta cells die off or otherwise become dysfunctional, cells in the person's body can't access free-circulating glucose, which accumulates in the bloodstream. The body is left to rely on fat stores rather than glucose for energy. Ketone bodies produced by fat burning make the blood more acidic, eventually leading to diabetic ketoacidosis (DKA).

As ketoacidosis progresses, the body tries to unload excess blood glucose through the kidneys. The undiagnosed person with T1D experiences incredible thirst and drinks fluids continuously and excessively. They pee away the day and night. Significant weight loss, hunger, and malaise follow. Hopefully, someone notices before the person slips into a coma and dies. A diagnosis is made after a trip to the doctor or emergency room.

Insulin therapy is restorative, so much so that when first widely available in 1922, it was viewed as a cure. Diabetes education follows. The person with T1D is informed that they can live a long and normal life *if* they eat a balanced, healthy diet *and* properly administer daily insulin delivered via pump or injection. However, this approach usually doesn't work very well. Most T1Ds live on a glycemic roller coaster, with many eventually experiencing significant complications. They may even plunge off the roller coaster and succumb from hypoglycemia or DKA long before a heart attack, stroke, or kidney failure kills them.

There are happy exceptions. Some people with T2D can reverse their metabolic syndromes through a healthy diet and exercise and thus eliminate their need for medication. Their blood sugars become normal, not because drugs, insulin, or both are driving them down, but because their metabolic processes have healed and are maintained in homeostasis while adequate pancreatic beta cell function remains. Some people with T1D survive for decades without significant complications. The famous Joslin Clinic in Boston awards a medal to fifty-year T1D survivors (see Figure 1.1).

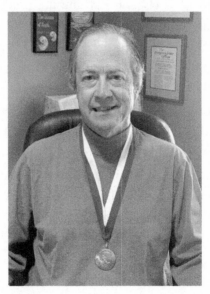

Figure 1.1. Chad and his medal. Fifty-four years and counting!

No One Size Fits All

Diabetes is complex. For example, obesity is not always a precursor to type 2 diabetes. The fact that 85 percent of those with T2D are overweight or obese means that 15 percent are not. In recent decades, children have been diagnosed with T2D, and 20 percent of American adolescents are now prediabetic.[8] There are now "double diabetics": obese, autoimmune people with T1D who have metabolic syndrome and insulin resistance. There is also an autoimmune variation of diabetes—latent autoimmune diabetes (LADA)—in which adults end up with the same treatment challenges as those with traditional T1D. Five novel subgroups of adult-onset diabetes were recently defined.[9] There is gestational diabetes that for many women eventually morphs into diabetes. Joslin Clinic researchers are among those who recently found that some persons with T1D still have insulin-producing beta cells that smooth disease management and prolong life expectancy. (A new sort of T1D?)

Different diabetes types and individual physiologic and metabolic differences determine the diabetes treatment protocols offered by care providers as well as the choices we must make about them. There are few pat definitions or answers across the board when managing the disease. For example, it would appear to be a no-brainer that you should eat a low-carbohydrate diet if you have diabetes. But even here, a special case allows for higher-carb eating for some (more on this in Chapter 5).

The Costs

Diabetes drives an unprecedented and costly health care crisis in the United States. As of 2017, almost one-third of all adult Americans either have diabetes or are prediabetic.[10] Only 10 percent of prediabetic people are even aware of their status, and according to one study, 70 percent of those who are prediabetic end up with the full-blown condition.[11] As impossible as it may sound, by 2040 one-third of all Americans could have diabetes; that's more than *100 million people* who will require diabetes-related medical care.

In 2017, diabetes cost the United States $327 billion—$237 billion in direct medical costs and another $90 billion in indirect costs, such as those associated with missed workdays or reduced productivity.[12] That's 25 percent of all health care costs.[13] At $16,750 per year, the average health care cost of each person with diabetes is more than *double* that of one who doesn't have the condition.[14] Of course, financial costs will grow along with new cases. Can you just imagine the individual and societal financial burden when one-third of us have diabetes?

And yet, this epidemiological disaster hasn't triggered front-page treatment. That's surprising. During the fourteenth century, approximately one-third of all Europeans died from the bubonic plague. It's not a big stretch to contemplate an American future where one-third of all deaths are tied, at least indirectly, to diabetes. True, those killed by the medieval plague died immediately, whereas physical decline typically occurs over many years with diabetes. (But at least those who died of the plague died quickly and not in wheelchairs, blinded, impotent, or gangrenous.) You can bet the citizens of medieval England were keenly focused on the Black Death. Why isn't there the same sense of urgency with the diabetes epidemic?

A similar analogy can be drawn to the COVID-19 disaster that struck the United States in early spring 2020. The country had to wreck its economy to slow or stop the pandemic's progress. Hundreds of millions of people masked up and practiced social distancing. That same level of attention to diabetes, *a condition that has and will continue to maim and kill many more people than COVID-19,* just isn't there.

Boatloads of dollars do go into diabetes-related medical care, but that's primarily for treatment. What about public policy directed at prevention and cure? Given the extent of the problem both now and in the near future, you'd expect the equivalent of the Manhattan Project that built the atom bomb, the NASA funding that put us on the moon, or the attention and resources paid to COVID-19. But it's not happening. For example, National Institutes of Health (NIH) funding is at almost three times more for HIV/AIDS research than for diabetes *despite more than 30 times more deaths* attributed to diabetes according to the same data set.[15] (But the actual difference is vastly greater; diabetes-related heart attack and stroke deaths aren't counted in this comparison.)

Part of the problem may be that diabetes devastation happens gradually. It's a slow-moving train wreck rather than a dramatically fast one like COVID-19. As with today's inattention to global warming, it's easily put aside by both sufferers and government policymakers. The problem has crept up at all levels. And the creeping continues.

The good news is that we don't have to rely on the government to save ourselves. In fact, given the inadequacies of the status quo, we *must* rely on ourselves. An important purpose of this book is to help you do this.

Questions for Your Care Providers

- *Why have I been diagnosed with diabetes? What type is it?*

- *What are possible diabetic complications and how might they be prevented?*

- *Am I experiencing complications?*

- *If so, what are they and how might I mitigate or reverse them?*

At this point, it's important to work with your care providers to become as knowledgeable as possible about your type of diabetes and its likely prognosis. From there, it's important to understand the treatment options you have, as well as the rationale for your current treatment.

Further Reading

BOOKS

The following two books represent conventional wisdom and standard practice. The first is a bit dated but still representative. Although the second is written for people with type 1 diabetes, there's a lot there for those with type 2.

- American Diabetes Association. *American Diabetes Association Complete Guide to Diabetes: The Ultimate Home Reference from the Diabetes Experts.* 5th ed. Arlington, VA: American Diabetes Association, 2011.

- Wood, Jamie, and Anne Peters. *The Type 1 Diabetes Self-Care Manual: A Complete Guide to Type 1 Diabetes across the Lifespan for People with Diabetes, Parents, and Caregivers.* Arlington, VA: American Diabetes Association, 2018.

The following book is an example of an integrative (sometimes referred to as "functional") medical approach to diabetes treatment. Integrative medical approaches combine practices and treatments from both traditional and alternative medical care.

- Morstein, Mona. *Master Your Diabetes: A Comprehensive, Integrative Approach for Both Type 1 and Type 2 Diabetes.* White River Junction, VT: Chelsea Green, 2017.

I recommend the following books for all people with diabetes.

- Bernstein, Richard K. *Dr. Bernstein's Diabetes Solution: The Complete Guide to Achieving Normal Blood Sugars.* 4th ed. New York: Little, Brown Spark, 2011.

- Brown, Adam. *Bright Spots and Landmines: The Diabetes Guide I Wish Someone Had Handed Me.* San Francisco: DiaTribe Foundation, 2017.

- Edelman, Steven V. (and Friends). *Taking Control of Your Diabetes.* 5th ed. West Islip, NY: Professional Communications, 2017.

- Fung, Jason. *The Diabetes Code: Prevent and Reverse Type 2 Diabetes Naturally.* Vancouver: Greystone Books, 2018. (This book is not just for those with T2D; it contains plenty of good stuff for people with T1D as well.)

- Greenberg, Riva. *Diabetes Do's and How-To's.* New York: SPI Management, 2013.

- Hirsch, James S. *Cheating Destiny: Living with Diabetes, America's Biggest Epidemic.* Boston: Houghton Mifflin, 2006.

- Ruhl, Jenny. *Blood Sugar 101: What They Don't Tell You about Diabetes.* 2nd ed. Turners Falls, MA: Technion Books, 2016.

For those who use a continuous glucose monitor (CGM) or are interested in close control with a glucometer, the following book is a great resource.

- Ponder, Stephen W., and Kevin L. McMahon. *Sugar Surfing: How to Manage Type 1 Diabetes in a Modern World.* Sausalito, CA: Mediself Press, 2015.

PERIODICALS

- *Diabetes Daily*: diabetesdaily.com

- *Diabetes Daily Grind*: diabetesdailygrind.com. (Check out the outstanding podcasts!)

- *Diabetes Forecast*: This was the ADA's flagship publication for those living with diabetes and their families. The ADA ceased the print publication in September 2020 but replaced it online with *Living Healthily*, at diabetes.org/healthy-living.

- *Diabetes Self-Management*: diabetesselfmanagement.com

- *ASweetLife*: asweetlife.org

- *Taking Control*: tcoyd.org/newsletter. This is the newsletter of the Taking Control of Your Diabetes (TCOYD) nonprofit organization.

BLOGS AND OTHER RESOURCES

Following are great sources of information and support.

- Beyond Type 1: beyondtype1.org

- Bezzy T2D: bezzyt2d.com

- *Diabetes Daily:* diabetesdaily.com

- *DiabetesMine:* healthline.com/diabetesmine

- *Diabetes Strong:* diabetesstrong.com

- *DiaTribe:* diatribe.org

- *Six Until Me:* sixuntilme.com/wp. Kerry Sparling ended her excellent blog, but its fourteen years of archives are worthwhile and still available.

For the best diabetes blogs for 2022 according to *eMedi-Health*, see Robert Floyd, "18 Best Diabetes Blogs to Help Manage Diabetes," *eMediHealth*, April 1, 2022, https://www.emedihealth.com/glands-hormones/diabetes/blogs-diabetes-management, and for a list of forums in general, see diatribe.org/diabetes-blogs-and-forums.

For mental health issues, a good reference is the ADA's *Mental Health Provider Directory*, found at professional.diabetes.org/ada-mental-health-provider-directory.

In-person conferences are an excellent way to get the latest and greatest from experts, to compare and contrast diabetes products on display, and to network with new friends with diabetes. The Taking Control of Your Diabetes (TCOYD) nonprofit organization (tcoyd.org/patient-events) does a great job with conferences. They have the top people in the diabetes world as presenters and host exhibits where you can learn about and compare and contrast all types of diabetes products and services. Conveners Drs.

Steve Edelman and Jeremy Pettus can be zany—for example, eating three donuts or three slices of pizza to check out insulin doses and blood sugar effects. Not something I do or recommend, but it's still instructive to watch (see tcoyd.org/2021/04/how -to-eat-three-donuts-and-stay-in-range and tcoyd.org/2021/10/ battle-of-the-blood-sugars-the-pizza-challenge). Dr. Pettus also plays a mean guitar!

Families with diabetic children might consider attending the annual Children with Diabetes Friends for Life conference (childrenwithdiabetes.com/conferences). It's truly one of the best places to learn and to connect on behalf of your child.

The following resources are helpful for insulin users from all over the world.

- Integrated Diabetes Services: integrateddiabetes.com. This education service is led by Gary Scheiner. In the United States, call 877-735-3648; outside the United States, call 001-610-642-6055.

- Saluté Nutrition: salutenutritionpllc.com. Led by Jennifer Okemah, this service offers online diabetes nutrition, counseling, and device training. In-person education is available in the Seattle, Washington, area. Call 425-285-5877.

- Dr. Jody Stanislaw: drjodynd.com. The services offered by Dr. Stanislaw include a private program, a free introductory call and sign-up (see drjodynd.com/consultation), online courses (see thriving-with-t1d.thinkific.com/collections), and a monthly T1D membership program (see the-type-1 -diabetes-crew.mn.co).

CHAPTER 2

THE HIERARCHY
OF DIABETES CARE

As It Is

People with diabetes hunger for answers because the traditional hierarchy of diabetes care has had a tough time delivering. You see this in judgmental self-help book titles—for example: *Take Control of Your Diabetes: The Essential Take-Charge Guide for Better Health and Better Living* (2009); *Blood Sugar 101: What They Don't Tell You about Diabetes* (2nd ed., 2016); *Bright Spots and Landmines: The Diabetes Guide I Wish Someone Had Handed Me* (2017); *Lies My Doctor Told Me: Medical Myths That Can Harm Your Health* (2017); and *Undoctored: Why Health Care Has Failed You and How You Can Become Smarter Than Your Doctor* (2017).

Dr. William Davis, the author of the last book, sums up the frustration in his introduction:

> The system is ready and willing to commit you to a life of taking drugs and injectable insulin for diabetes, dealing with the eventual heart disease, kidney failure, and peripheral neuropathy with more drugs and procedures, providing "education" designed by people who put commercial interests first, while no one provides the handful of inexpensive health strategies that have been shown to reduce, even fully reverse, type 2 diabetes.[1]

Dr. Davis is talking about nutrition and exercise when he refers to "inexpensive health strategies." This combination effectively addresses most T2D conditions. Significant weight reduction could eliminate—or at least significantly reduce—the need for medication for the 85 percent of people with T2D who are overweight or obese with associated metabolic syndrome.

Books promising reversal or cure of diabetes for those with T2D are based on this premise. There's a lot of them. Just in my local Camano Island, Washington, library system, I found thirty-five titles promising a cure, the reversal, or the end of diabetes via nutrition and exercise—about 10 percent of the diabetes books on the shelves.

DRUGS AND DEVICES

So, if nutrition and exercise are so darned important, why are drugs and devices the very foundation of the current hierarchy of diabetes care (Figure 2.1)?

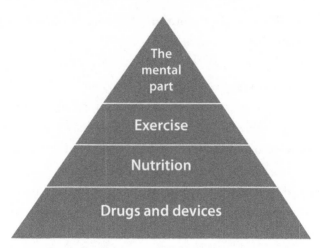

Figure 2.1. The current hierarchy of diabetes care.

There are many reasons. For starters, few traditional family practitioners are trained in diabetes, much less nutrition. Less than 4 percent of education time in medical school is spent on diabetes, and nutrition may be covered only in passing, if at all.[2] A survey of accredited US medical schools between 2008 and 2009 found that only 25 percent provided a nutrition course, down from 30 percent just a few years earlier.[3] And 90 percent of surveyed cardiologists reported receiving little or no nutrition education during their fellowship training. And yet 95 percent of this sample believed that their role includes personally providing basic nutrition information to patients.

This is as it should be, particularly given the close connection between diabetes and cardiovascular disease, but as the study concluded, "Nutritional interventions are the foundation of clinical care guidelines, yet cardiovascular specialists lack the nutrition education to effectively implement these guidelines."[4]

Conventional practitioners and their patients also believe in the efficacy of drugs and devices. We're used to the idea—even expect—that medical miracles such as organ transplants, vaccines, antibiotics, and pills of all varieties will fix our ailments. Diabetes medications and devices are part of this mix and the associated expectation.

Big Pharma has worked overtime to develop blood sugar-influencing pharmaceuticals, including still more insulins. Devices have come along to help in the process: for example, glucometers in the 1980s and continuous glucose monitors (CGM) in the early 2000s. Current hybrid insulin-delivery systems still require mealtime boluses from the user, but a true closed-loop artificial pancreas that can do this is in the works. The 2020 ADA consumer guide published in *Diabetes Forecast* touts *more than 240* meters, CGMs, pumps, meds, and more on its cover. That's a big number. What's even more remarkable is that the 2018 consumer guide listed only 150-plus products. *A 60 percent increase in just two years!*

These medical miracles reinforce the notion that those with diabetes can just go to the doctor and get medicine or a gadget to fix blood sugar, much like having a broken bone set or taking prescription antibiotics to clear up a sinus infection. Too bad it's not that simple with diabetes!

Underlying philosophy also figures in. Nontraditional medical practitioners claim that conventional medicine is allopathic, focusing on drugs and devices rather than properly—and preventatively—holistically treating the body over time. Their position is that traditional physicians have blinders on and just want to write scripts. A study did find that 76 percent of office visits for type 2 diabetes result in a prescription.[5]

However, even if conventional care providers possessed what some view as enlightened knowledge, the fifteen- or twenty-minute assembly line office visit leaves little time for extensive counseling. Even if there was time, conventional physicians and other care providers usually aren't trained to help the patient do little more than simply cope. (The Flourishing Treatment Approach [FTA], developed by Riva Greenberg and Boudewijn Bertsch, may help move this needle.[6])

So the physician interviews the patient, looks at a screen, analyzes metrics, and after consultation, makes a drug or device modification or recommendation. Then, it's on to the next patient. Nutritional counseling tends to be shuttled off to workshops or sessions with nutritionists, dietitians, or diabetes care and education specialists (DCESes) with mixed results.

NUTRITION

Good, useful information can be gained from nutrition workshops and sessions, but then we're told something like this: "A low-fat, low-sugar, high-protein diet with plenty of fruits, vegetables, and whole grains is the best dietary prescription for keeping blood sugar in check."[7] This advice might be good for a person with T2D who has some pancreatic beta cell function, particularly relative to the cheeseburgers, fries, milkshakes, and pizza they've been eating. But if you're completely insulin-dependent, consuming "plenty" of fruits and whole grains to keep blood sugar in check can be tough. Vegetables like corn, carrots, and beets are loaded with sugar. There can be more sugar in a banana than in a Hershey's chocolate bar, more in two slices of whole-grain bread than in a Snickers bar.

I've attended numerous nutrition workshops and sessions over the years. Not once have I heard an informed variation from traditional "healthy eating." For example, the roving nutritionist at a 2018 Taking Control of Your Diabetes (TCOYD) conference for those with T1D told me she had never heard of *Dr. Bernstein's Diabetes Solution*, the bible of the low-carb movement; nor was she aware of low-carb eating as an alternative to MyPlate.*

MyPlate is not necessarily wrong or bad for some of us, as I explain in a later chapter, but the diet should be followed cautiously. A newspaper columnist describes the problem with MyPlate this way: "MyPlate is based on the concept that every meal should be made up of half fruits and vegetables. But the USDA considers potatoes, corn, and frozen juice concentrate as produce. Luckily, none of us are diabetic."[8]

Just recently, the ADA spun off MyPlate with the Diabetes Plate Method. Fill half of your plate with low-carb vegetables, a quarter with lean protein, the other quarter with starchy carbs, and drink water or a low-carb beverage.[9] This approach is more diabetes-friendly than MyPlate, but it's contradictory in the sense that the organization asserts elsewhere that no one diabetes diet is best.[10]

Before the Diabetes Plate Method came along, the ADA also equivocated when it listed seven different diet choices on its website: Mediterranean, vegetarian or vegan, low- and very low-carbohydrate, low-fat, very low-fat, DASH, and Paleo. Likewise, at the turn of the twenty-first century, the organization moved from a ban on high-sugar foods to dietary moderation rather than deprivation.[11]

---

* MyPlate is published by the US Department of Agriculture Center for Nutrition Policy and Promotion. It depicts a place setting with a plate and glass divided into five food groups: fruits, grains, vegetables, protein, and dairy. It replaced the USDA's Food Guide Pyramid in 2011, ending almost two decades of the traditional food pyramid that listed carbs as the foundation of "healthy" eating.

And still more flip-flopping from the ADA can be seen in articles in the organization's past flagship consumer magazine, *Diabetes Forecast*. The titles of the articles "The Carbohydrate Craze" (May–June 2017) and "The Keto Craze" (January–February 2019) were changed when they were moved online to "Navigating a Low-Carb Eating Plan" and "What You Need to Know about the Ketogenic Diet," respectively. Removing "craze" from the titles eliminated bias that shouldn't have been there in the first place. Paradoxically, the articles were still well balanced even with "craze" in the initial titles.

It's not surprising that the ADA wrestles with diabetic nutrition. This also occurs in trade books and popular literature. For example, Dr. George King, a physician and the chief scientific officer for the Joslin Clinic, claims that his plant-based diet of 70 percent carbs will reverse type 2 diabetes in twelve weeks.[12] The aforementioned Dr. Bernstein, also a physician, claims success with a ketogenic, high-fat diet that's less than 10 percent carbohydrates.[13] There couldn't be a greater disparity between two diets recommended by bona fide diabetes experts that both promise positive results.

In Chapter 5, I address the diabetes dietary controversy with a framework and standards that reconcile disparate views and cover not just the *what* but also the *why* of healthy diabetes eating. Of course, my chapter will not be the last word on the subject!

EXERCISE

Moving on now to exercise (no wordplay intended!).

This subject might be covered by a physician in an office visit with a few minutes of "eat less, move more" advice and maybe a referral to an exercise physiologist or a trainer. Join the YMCA. Find a physical activity you enjoy. Go for a daily walk. There's little else that the health care provider can do. Physicians and DCESes usually don't have sufficient training to advise patients on the subject. There's also a fundamental problem with how the nature and purpose of exercise are typically covered. Chapter 7 covers the topic, but a quick hint—you don't have to like doing it, and you don't need a lot of it to get real benefit.

THE MENTAL PART

Finally, the mental part. This is the least emphasized area in the current hierarchy of diabetes care. It typically starts with training. Initially, this involves fifteen to twenty hours of diabetes education led by a DCES, though a training visit might also occur for those whose diabetes life begins in the hospital. The newly diagnosed learn the importance of counting carbs, exercising regularly, and following a "healthier" diet, usually some variation of MyPlate or the Mediterranean Diet. Special sessions for insulin pump or continuous glucose monitoring (CGM) training may also be involved. A lot of ground to cover in a short amount of time!

Subsequently, care providers may not have the time or the expertise to do much counseling, so eventually they might refer patients to a diabetes support group. Almost all large medical practices and hospitals have group therapy or sessions available, usually led by a DCES. In these sessions, people with diabetes share the challenges of daily living and learn from one another and the DCES. Much information is shared online as well, through social media and blogs such as those listed at the end of Chapter 1. Individual sessions with a DCES might be arranged. Occasionally, a behavioral counselor might be recommended.

Beyond local efforts to address diabetes-related mental health issues, there's the Behavioral Diabetes Institute (founded by Dr. William Polonsky) and the Center for Diabetes and Mental Health (founded by Dr. Mark Heyman), both located in San Diego.

Dr. Polonsky is a clinical psychologist and is considered the nation's leader in all things behavioral and emotional relating to diabetes. His classic book *Diabetes Burnout: What to Do When You Can't Take It Anymore*, published twenty years ago by the ADA, has good information that still applies today.

A spin on burnout, not covered in the book but developed later by Dr. Polonsky and his associates, is the current hot topic of diabetes distress—distress caused by the relentless pressure of medical bills, managing complex medications, "diet police" family members, coping with denial, and worrying about and dealing with physical complications, both short- and long-term, without ever having a break. This distress may not rise to the level of clinical depression but is intertwined with depression when it occurs and is diagnosed.[14] You can even assess your distress by completing a standardized instrument, the Diabetes Distress Scale (DDS), developed by Dr. Polonsky and his associates (see diabetesdistress.org/take-dd-survey).

Dr. Heyman's approach to diabetes distress centers around five tools for becoming mentally "unstuck": diabetes education, support, mindfulness, self-compassion, and gratitude. These tools focus on being in the present, not beating yourself up for the occasional blood sugar misstep, and even being grateful for the silver lining that diabetes can offer (for example, the benefits of eating and exercising more healthily).[15]

There's more on diabetes distress offered elsewhere: Don't try to be perfect, be sure to talk about your feelings, learn to cope with guilt, and know when you are especially vulnerable.[16] Through all conceptions on diabetes distress is the common thread of the importance of reaching out to others.

All well and good, but dealing with distress with measures such as self-compassion, talking about your feelings, and reaching out to others are little more than Band-Aids if an inappropriate diet, the mistaken belief that medication can effectively "cover" that diet, and inadequate exercise *are not also addressed*. Doesn't it make sense to also focus on the causes of distress rather than just treat the symptoms or outcomes?

Not to put too fine of a point on it, but there's another disease that shares much in common with diabetes and also causes great distress. As with diabetes, sufferers contend with a chronic condition involving denial and adverse consequences. Family members are similarly affected and police the sufferer's behavior. The disease is also progressive. This disease, like diabetes, usually ends in debilitation and death if not arrested with a twelve-step program or other intervention. I'm talking here about alcoholism. (I cover the benefits of a twelve-step perspective in managing diabetes in Chapter 4.)

An alcoholic must quit drinking. That's their only solution. We can't quit eating. *But we can still change the way we think about food* and, from this baseline, *change what we eat*. We can also *change the way we think about exercise* and build a manageable modicum of it into our lives. That's addressing the cause, not just treating symptoms of distress, and it's the basis of the mental part of the hierarchy of diabetes care—as it should be.

As It Should Be

The mental part should come first, not last, because it sets the stage for all that follows (see Figure 2.2). Accurate information about the disease from care providers is just a starting point. From there, we need to acknowledge that *our metabolism isn't normal*. We have a disease. Treating this disease requires a permanent change in our relationship with food—its role in our lives and the *why* and *what* behind our eating. It also requires rethinking and changing our relationship with exercise.

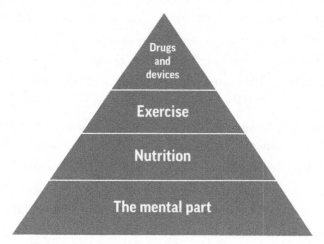

Figure 2.2. The hierarchy of diabetes care, as it should be.

Get this part right, and the consequent need for drugs and devices is minimized. For most people with T2D, the goal is to safely manage blood sugar with diet and exercise alone. Those with T1D can pursue the goal of doing the same, requiring as little insulin as possible. A stable glycemic merry-go-round replaces the sometimes-terrifying glycemic roller coaster. Stress associated with hypoglycemic and hyperglycemic excursions as well as actual or prospective long-term complications of retinopathy, neuropathy, nephropathy, cardiovascular disease, and the like is reduced. Diabetes-related burnout, distress, and depression retreat to the background, maybe even becoming nonissues.

The balance of this book moves through the hierarchy of diabetes care as it should be. The next two chapters address the mental part after orientation when a newly diagnosed person with diabetes, in consultation with their care providers, ponders how to adapt and live healthily. These chapters also apply to frustrated long-termers who know something is wrong but can't pin it down.

From there, I move up the hierarchy to nutrition and exercise and then to what should be the least-emphasized topic in the hierarchy—drugs and devices.[†] A final chapter shows how all these pieces work together in a healthy diabetes life.

Riva Greenberg Weighs in on Diabetes and Its Treatment

Chad's email arrived in my inbox as a total surprise. I didn't know him, but I was immediately impressed that he's lived with type 1 diabetes even longer than my fifty years. He

continued

---

† Insulin is lifesaving and sustaining for those with T1D, but it's included in what should be the least-emphasized category because relying on insulin (and other diabetes medications), in the absence of an effective mental frame, nutrition, and exercise, contributes to poor outcomes.

shared that he was writing this book and invited me to be a part of it.

While I don't agree with some of Chad's thinking, I do agree with much of it—especially its impact to help "people with diabetes" (PWD) live our healthiest and happiest lives.

As Chad does, I believe that diabetes is a condition of carbohydrate intolerance and that we can better manage our blood sugar with carbohydrate reduction. I eat low carb and have for years. It keeps my blood sugar off the "roller coaster" and increases my time in range. The remarkable thing is that I don't miss those carb-loaded bagels and scones I used to eat every day. We know taste buds can change in just a few weeks.

Once, over brunch with acquaintances with type 1 diabetes, a woman yelled at me while buttering her bagel, "Don't expect me to make such sacrifices!" But my life is not about sacrifices and not without goodies. I bake my own scones and biscotti, and I even make pizza dough with almond flour. I enjoy pasta made from soybeans and lentils, and my husband is not disappointed. If they shipped me off to a desert island with just three items—plain yogurt, almond butter, and a pan of roasted vegetables with olive oil—I wouldn't feel deprived.

I also agree on the value of exercise for overall health, weight maintenance, the psychological boost, and insulin sensitivity. I walk an hour almost every day, and when I have to miss it for a few days, my body needs more insulin. However, I'm not for a "grin and bear it" attitude toward exercise. If that works for you, more power to you. But if you're like us creatures of comfort, I believe doing something you like has more sticking power. Throughout my years with diabetes, I have tried weightlifting, working with a personal trainer, running, yoga, ping-pong, tennis— and yet, all fell by the wayside.

I started walking forty years ago when the subways in Manhattan went on strike. Hundreds of us laced up our sneakers and walked to and from work. I did it for a few months out of necessity, and for the next forty years out of enjoyment and a sense of accomplishment. These days, I listen to a podcast during my walk, so if I miss a walk, I really miss my podcast. Low-carb eating and walking are how I've dropped thirty-five pounds over the years and kept them off just as long.

A HUMAN-ORIENTED APPROACH

After nineteen years of working in diabetes, over the last few, I've been sharing with health care professionals (HCPs) around the world a different way of working with people who have diabetes. It's an approach I designed called the Flourishing Approach.[17] Rather than "fixing problems" with the goal of avoiding complications, it helps people identify and build on what they're doing well, see more of what is possible, and aim to achieve their best health.

The conventional treatment approach is similar to that used for acute conditions: treating the body, not the person. The Flourishing Approach, conversely, treats the whole human being. It's grounded in the understanding that we

33 *continued*

are sociobiological creatures who require safety and belonging to flourish. It uses insights from neurobiology, as well as how people create health and resilience and grow from adversity. As such, it fosters trust and psychological safety between PWDs and HCPs.

This alchemy calms the nervous system, which allows you to hear better, think more clearly and creatively, and see new solutions when you visit your doctor. "Doing diabetes" without a sense of partnership is, for patients and practitioners alike, like running a three-legged race.

Here are steps you can take to move in the direction of flourishing:

1. Learn everything you can.

2. Appreciate what you do well. Think, *How do I do it? How might I do just a bit more of it?*

3. Reflect on one positive thing that diabetes has given you. Some positives I've heard include the joy of helping family members with diabetes, a sense of humility, pride at losing weight and keeping it off, becoming healthier, developing new friendships, and feeling closer to a partner.

4. Tell your HCP what you'd like to work on next and brainstorm together how to do that.

5. Ask your HCP to repeat anything you didn't hear or understand.

COMPLEXITY AND MASTERY OF BLOOD SUGAR

The Flourishing Approach also acknowledges that managing diabetes and blood sugar is complex; it's not a simple cause-and-effect ("do this and that will happen") as health professionals have been trained to think. This complexity comes from the many variables that affect blood sugar—known and unknown, certain and unpredictable, interwoven and separate, obvious and hidden, and inside and outside our body. This means we cannot "control" our blood sugar. Instead, we daily—often hourly—must make sense of it and decide what to do next. I point this out in a chapter I wrote, "When Disease Requires a Complexity Framework."[18]

Because many HCPs believe that our salvation lies in controlling our blood sugar, which is something we cannot do, many people with diabetes see themselves as failures. And, as Chad also notes in Chapter 3, some give up their management entirely. When I share this complexity knowledge with others with diabetes, they feel liberated. Our best effort is made not by trying to control blood sugar, but by gaining the skills to navigate blood sugar.

Navigating means:

1. Knowing how to influence your blood sugar to best prevent highs and lows

2. Recognizing blood sugar patterns—for example, being more insulin-resistant in the morning—and knowing how to nudge blood sugar into the desired target range no matter what the number is

continued

I also believe that the complexity of managing diabetes and life defies prioritizing management domains as Chad's pyramid suggests. And just as with YDMV (your diabetes may vary), what may be my most pressing issue may not be yours. Working from a complexity mindset, we benefit instead from seeing the management tiers in a flow state and working with what's most critical in the moment, and from a space of potentiality, with whatever may emerge.

LOOKING BACK AND FORWARD

Flourishing for me includes a healthy dose of historical gratitude. Getting T1D at the age of eighteen in 1972 was ten years before glucose meters came out. I was told to take one shot of insulin a day at 8:00 a.m., and my "diabetes diet" translated into "don't eat candy bars"! I'm grateful for all the advances that help me, such as my continuous glucose monitor; faster, small glucose meters; insulins that don't peak; and sharper, thinner needles.

Casting my eyes forward on diabetes treatment, I'd like to see the onus on self-efficacy, the work we load on a patient's shoulders lightened by social efficacy, and having government and business leaders participate in making healthy choices and activities easier and more accessible.

Here are some questions you can ask your HCP to move from coping to flourishing with diabetes:

1. Ask your burning question not when your hand is on the doorknob to leave, but early on.

2. What am I doing well? (This helps you both talk about improvement rather than fixing a problem.)

3. What one small step do you think will improve my management?

4. Can I have a referral for Diabetes Self-Management Education and Support (DSMES) services?

.   .   .

Riva Greenberg is a health researcher, health coach, corporate advisor, author, and inspirational speaker. Having lived with type 1 diabetes for more than fifty years, her work is dedicated to helping people with diabetes and health professionals work collaboratively in a way that helps both to flourish. Riva has written three books: *Diabetes Do's and How-To's*, *50 Diabetes Myths That Can Ruin Your Life and the 50 Diabetes Truths That Can Save It*, and *The ABCs of Loving Yourself with Diabetes*, as well as hundreds of articles and blog posts at Diabetes Stories. Riva is working with the Centers for Disease Control and Prevention to brand DSMES, is a member of a global diabetes experts forum (Controversies in Obesity, Diabetes, and Hypertension, codhyglobalexpertsforum.com), was an A1C Champion peer mentor for ten years, has spoken at the World Health Organization, and is recognized for her humanistic work by professional associations and organizations.

Questions for Your Care Providers

To the questions Ms. Greenberg raised in her commentary, I add the following for your care providers. (Please note that more specific questions for care providers on the subjects of the mental part, nutrition, and exercise appear later after chapters on those subjects.)

- *What are your views of healthy nutrition for people with diabetes?*

- *How can I learn more about the subject?* These first two questions apply to all members of your team—the physician, DCES, and nutritionist. The answers will uncover biases and shed light on the extent to which your caregivers can provide useful information on nutrition. For example, a DCES trained as a registered nurse, one with a master's degree in social work, or a conventionally trained physician may have zero expertise in nutrition. Depending on the nature of your diabetes or general health, a nutritionist trained years ago who only has an unmodified MyPlate or Mediterranean Diet to suggest may have little to offer you.

- *What are your views and advice on exercise?*

- *What local mental health care resources can you recommend?* (Ask this question especially if you're feeling distressed or depressed.)

- *Is there a local diabetes support group I might join?*

Further Reading

BOOKS

- Davis, William. *Undoctored: Why Health Care Has Failed You and How You Can Become Smarter Than Your Doctor.* New York: Rodale Books, 2017.

- Heyman, Mark. *Diabetes Sucks and You Can Handle It: Your Guide to Managing the Emotional Challenges of T1D.* Eugene, OR: Luminare Press, 2022. (The book is good for T2Ds as well!)

- Polonsky, William H. *Diabetes Burnout: What to Do When You Can't Take It Anymore.* Alexandria, VA: American Diabetes Association, 1999.

- Rosman, Paul, and David Edelman. *Thriving with Diabetes: Learn How to Take Charge of Your Body to Balance Your Sugars and Improve Your Lifelong Health.* Beverly, MA: Fair Winds Press, 2015. (Chapters 10, 11, and 12 provide excellent coverage of the mental part of diabetes.)

- Vieira, Ginger. *Dealing with Diabetes Burnout: How to Recharge and Get Back on Track When You Feel Frustrated and Overwhelmed Living with Diabetes.* New York: Demos Medical, 2014.

OTHER RESOURCES

- Dr. Mark Heyman's website: thediabetespsychologist.com

CHAPTER 3

THE MENTAL PART: GETTING BACK TO BASICS

G etting the mental part right requires challenging and changing your diet status quo, beginning with your assumptions about food. A framework for living one day at a time based on a healthier eating pattern (with exercise) then needs to follow. But first, a few words about motivation.

Motivation

A useful concept for understanding motivation related to diabetes is Victor Vroom's Expectancy Theory.[1] According to Vroom, motivation is driven by the belief that effort will lead to performance (expectancy), the belief that performance will lead to an outcome (instrumentality), and the value placed on the outcome (valence). The relationship among the parts is multiplicative. If any of the factors is low, the force of motivation will be low.

For example, I may have little faith that my 50 percent-carb MyPlate diet with occasional treats will lead to acceptable blood sugars because I just can't seem to get off the glycemic roller coaster. Consequently, my expectancy—the belief that effort will lead to performance—on a scale of zero to 100 percent is low at 20 percent. However, instrumentality is high at 100 percent because I fully believe that in-range, stable, average blood sugars are instrumental to reducing complications, an outcome that is possible based on the research, most notably the famous 1992 Diabetes Control and Complications Trial (DCCT).[2] Valence is also high at 100 percent because I truly value the outcome of a long, less-distressing, complication-free life.

Despite my strong instrumentality and valence levels, my force of motivation is still low (20% × 100% × 100% = only 20%, just one-fifth of my total motivation possible). That's because my initial belief that my efforts will lead to the performance of successfully controlling diabetes is too low. I'm defeated from the start. I just can't do it. I may even give up and eat whatever I want. In the judgmental language of some care providers, I become noncompliant.

I've seen this pattern repeatedly. My friends with diabetes don't want to resign themselves to defeat, but accurately matching medication to their poor diets seems impossible. Allowable treats or exceptions to the rule add to the chaos. You know— "I'll just have diabetic desserts or eat pasta just twice a week." But they can't get off the roller coaster. They may stop checking blood sugars or take a blasé approach to medication (or both).

"I'll have the pumpkin pie; I'll just inject more insulin," they say. My friends erroneously think the key to success is balancing medication and large amounts of carbs ingested through "normal eating." They might go back to their doctor, who will change or add medication.

However, covering food with medication isn't like tuning a piano. There are just too many moving parts. Even if my friends hit the nail on the head by perfectly matching medication with carbs, there are still *forty-one other factors* affecting their blood sugar in play, such as protein and fat consumption with a meal, stress levels, exercise before eating, illness, how much sleep they got the night before, and the "dawn phenomenon" in the morning when hormones elevate blood sugar.[3] It's all overwhelming, frustrating, and demotivating.

People with diabetes can only improve their belief that efforts will lead to a positive performance—and thus improve their motivation—if they adopt a dietary regimen that can be realistically controlled and managed. Otherwise, they're set up to fail. *This means simplifying and getting back to basics*—going old-school by reducing carbs (for most of us), avoiding sugar (for all of us), not overeating protein, and just generally eating differently than what is considered normal.

Normal eating isn't in the cards for those of us with diabetes, despite what some experts may have us believe. We need to get this part right. A rationale for doing so follows.

The "People with Diabetes Can't Eat Sugar Is a Myth" Myth

The standard normal American diet includes eating sugar, sometimes a lot of it. But should we really eat the stuff? A 2018 expert's quote from a magazine titled *Living Well with Diabetes* says it's okay:

> Today, it's easier than ever for people with diabetes to live in our sugar-saturated world. The notion that sugar is off-limits is an outdated myth. "People with diabetes are often surprised that sugar isn't a forbidden food," says Mark Peterson, vice president of medical information for the American Diabetes Association. "They just have to account for it in their overall eating plan."[4]

A Joslin Clinic expert also says it's a myth that those with diabetes can't eat sugar.[5] Eating or drinking sugar is okay if we just don't overdo it. This claim comes from a diabetes magazine titled *Outsmart Diabetes*. (Eating sugar is now part of outsmarting diabetes?) Professor David Nathan, MD, director of the Diabetes Center at Massachusetts General Hospital, says completely avoiding sugar is "unrealistic, unpalatable, and unsustainable."[6]

The sugary frosting on this proverbial cake is the ADA's current position that sugar is okay for us—no different than any other carbohydrate in a responsible eating plan. We just need to account for it.

Baloney! What experts are telling us—that it's a myth we can't eat sugar—is itself a myth. Doing so just doesn't make sense.

Saying it's a myth that we can't eat sugar is like saying it's a myth that alcoholics can't drink alcohol. A drink a week, drinking in moderation, or drinking for special occasions is okay. Just account for the alcohol you're drinking, and don't overdo it. You know, drink beer rather than vodka, and don't do it every day. That's not going to work any better for an alcoholic than is telling a middle-aged overweight or obese person with T2D with a lifetime of bad eating habits that they can continue to eat sugar or telling a person with T1D they can eat regularly eat pie and cake just by adding more insulin.

Glucose, the simplest sugar, is what all carbohydrates other than fiber ultimately become in the body, whether their starting point is carbs from a potato, an apple, a glass of milk, or a teaspoon of table sugar in a cup of coffee. Types of sugar in reasonable quantities, such as the lactose in milk and fructose in fruit, have always been part of healthy eating for some of us and everyone else. However, when diabetes experts and the ADA say sugar is no longer off-limits, they're really making a special case in favor of sucrose (table sugar), a combination of fructose and glucose, and the high-fructose corn syrup contained in many processed foods. One is not healthier or better than the other, and both are bad for us.

To return to the analogy of the alcoholic, how many readers know of a person with a drinking problem who tried to cut back? For example, just drinking on weekends or special occasions (unsuccessfully)? If not cutting back, how about the alcoholic who switches to beer or wine instead of the hard stuff (unsuccessfully)? It's well-established in the literature that alcoholics need to stop drinking. The situation with added sugar is no different for people with diabetes, particularly the majority who are overweight or obese from a lifetime of sugar-drenched eating habits. Giving a green light means that the pleasurable serotonin brain rush of sugar always beckons.

Perhaps the comparison to alcoholism is invalid. After all, alcohol is addictive and sugar isn't—or is it? Sugar's addictiveness is up for debate. It's powerful stuff. One study famously found that lab rats given a choice between cocaine and sugar chose the sugar *94 percent of the time!*[7] I realize that humans aren't rats and this was only one study, but the point is still apropos. Sugar is seductive. It's not surprising that researchers have concluded that "the same neurobiological pathways that are implicated in drug abuse also modulate food consumption."[8]

The food reward associated with sugar is especially pronounced when combined in a deadly duo with dietary fat, as is the case with fast food and desserts. Obesity and addiction researcher Dr. Stephen Guyenet observes:

> Foods that are skillful combinations of fat, sugar, starch, salt, and delightful flavors likely cause your brain to release high levels of dopamine, sometimes provoking addiction in susceptible people. And when a person excludes a problem food for a long time, then suddenly has it in front of them at the dinner table, those latent craving pathways are reactivated—just as they are for drugs.[9]

Thinking it's okay to eat sugar also sets up a slippery slope. If the doctor or nutritionist says to us, "Eat a healthy diet," and that healthy diet includes sugar, then how much is too much? Is jelly on morning toast okay, since that's not overdoing it and it's been accounted for and covered by medication? Same with Pop-Tarts, since we don't eat them every morning and can cover them with medication? Is it okay now to eat apple pie because a smaller piece is being covered—an eighth of a pie rather than the quarter of a pie that used to be eaten? By the same reasoning, ice cream and chocolate cake are now okay, especially if just for special occasions. I could go on.

The American Heart Association says it's unhealthy to eat more than six teaspoons of added sugar daily for women and nine for men, but in the real world, the average American eats two to three times this amount—about sixty-six pounds of added sugar per year and nineteen teaspoons *per day*. I'm talking here about *added* sugar in goodies, on cereal, or in a cup of coffee, not the fructose in fruit or lactose in milk.[10] This is the poisoned dietary sea that the newly diagnosed person with diabetes has been swimming in. And now some experts expect this person to finesse sugar consumption to a still supposedly healthy place? To have their sugary cake and eat it too?

This expectation doesn't make sense. The slope is too slippery. We need to conscientiously avoid sugar, especially in the form of sucrose or the high-fructose corn syrup added to most processed foods and sodas. Eating added sugar is certainly palatable for us but doing so is not realistic or sustainable (for life).

Desserts and Fast Food Are Okay Too?

Even desserts are okay? It appears so. There are diabetes dessert recipe books, and diabetes periodicals often include images of decadent goodies on the cover and in dessert sections. For example, the cover of the August 2017 *Diabetes Self-Management* exclaimed, "Yes! You can have strawberry shortcake" and "One sweet summer!" over a luscious graphic of strawberry shortcake with whipped cream. I'm not cherry-picking. I Googled "diabetes dessert recipe books" and came back with 12.9 million hits!

These desserts typically contain more than one-third of all the daily carbs a healthy lower-carbohydrate diet should have. And that's just dessert. For just one meal.

What about fast food? After all, over one-third of the US population eats at least one fast-food meal daily.[11] Why not us too? Some diabetes experts think we should be included. For example, at the nutrition breakout session at the 2018 Taking

Control of Your Diabetes (TCOYD) conference, the nutritionist asked carb counters to raise their hands. Just about every hand went up. She later showed us how to count carbs using the example of a Burger King Single Whopper versus a Double Whopper!

Many years ago, at a seminar for insulin pump users sponsored by the manufacturer Medtronic, the DCES presenter showed a crowd of people with diabetes, including me, how to use the magic of dual-wave-pumping technology to cover *pizza*!

The underlying logic in play is that even bad food can be successfully covered through the modern-day miracle of diabetes drugs and devices. However, this is fallacious thinking. As a person with T1D, try successfully covering 100 carb grams with insulin after eating a high-fat Taco Bell, Pizza Hut, KFC, or McDonald's meal and then contending with the forty-one other potential factors affecting blood sugar (including protein conversion to glucose through gluconeogenesis and insulin resistance from dietary fat), and you'll see what I mean. Ditto if you're someone with T2D consuming fast food daily who's tried to control blood sugar with diet, exercise, and the drug metformin. It doesn't work.

To the expert claim that "You can have it!," I have to say, "No, you can't (or shouldn't)." Because you have diabetes. Your metabolism isn't normal.

The Fallacy of Normalcy

Figure 3.1 is the diary of person with T1D that shows food and insulin boluses. This fellow eats a small piece of chocolate cake when no one is watching and loves butterscotch pudding. Trix cereal, a breakfast favorite, requires a bolus of 12 units. This person also injects large boluses to cover foods such as pasta, pancakes, three large slices of pizza, and a large bowl of ice cream. All this is an example of the fallacy of normalcy—the mistaken

Usual Meals	Usual Rapid-Acting Insulin Dose[a]
Breakfast	
Just coffee with milk (no food)	3 units
Bagel with cream cheese	10 units
Bowl of cold cereal with milk *(I love Trix!)*	12 units
Bowl of hot cereal (no milk)	7 units
Pancakes or French toast	15 units
Scrambled eggs (2) with buttered toast (1 slice)	6 units
English muffin with peanut butter	3.5 units
Lunch	
Tuna, turkey, or veggie sandwich	10 units
Veggie burger	12 units
Soup and salad	8 units
Dinner	
Typical pasta dinner	14 units
Large salad with fresh bread	10 units
Chicken, fish, or meat dinner	12 units
3 Large slices of pizza	18 units

Unusual Meals

Restaurants

Usually add 5 to 10 units to my normal dose because I always find myself eating more in a restaurant than I do at home

Desserts (Yes, I do eat desserts once in awhile!)	
Small scoop of ice cream	3 units
Large bowl of ice cream	8 units
Cookies (2 or 3)	5 to 7 units
Small piece of chocolate cake *(when no one is watching me)*	6 to 8 units
Pudding (I love butterscotch)	4 to 5 units

[a] These doses are my usual normal premeal dose of Apidra, Humalog, or Novolog.

Figure 3.1. Food diary of a person with T1D. (From S. V. Edelman, *Taking Control of Your Diabetes*, 5th ed. [West Islip, NY: Professional Communications, 2017]. Reprinted by permission from Taking Control of Your Diabetes [tcoyd .org], a 501(c)3 organization.)

belief that we should and can eat like everyone else, all thanks to the miracle of drugs and devices.

According to the book where his diary appears, this person has complications after battling TD1 for over forty years. He is also an endocrinologist and a highly successful, respected member of the diabetes establishment (as he should be). I respectfully disagree with his food choices. You can too.

Another example of the fallacy of normalcy concerns sushi. You should think of sushi as table sugar wrapped in seaweed; it comes in at about 8 carb grams *per bite*. The culprit is its polished white rice, a food that is close to pure glucose on the glycemic index. A nutritionist in an organization led by a diabetes guru who is truly one of the best diabetes minds in America advocates a "sushi hack" for us. In computer parlance, a hack is a workaround. In this case, we are advised to cover 30 carb grams with insulin *before we even sit down in the restaurant*.[12] That's just a starting point. More carbs to cover will come with this meal.

A hack? Because we want to eat sushi like a person with a healthy metabolism? I respectfully disagree with this thinking as well. So can you. In the case of this expert, he laments in another column his struggles with control, confessing his A1cs had crept up close to 8 percent, an unhealthy average blood sugar north of 180 mg/dl.[13]

There's no intent here to ambush people I greatly admire who have given so much to the diabetes community. It's just that "normal eating" shouldn't be in the cards for us if we want to be healthy. That's just the way it is.

A final example comes from a summer 2019 conference on type 1 diabetes convened by a diabetes organization in the Pacific Northwest. I enjoyed the conference. The hard part, though, was the food. Lunch included choices of big pieces of bread for big sandwiches and pasta salad loaded with fat. Full-octane cookies were included in an afternoon snack. It was Mexican food for a dinner buffet: flour tortillas, enchiladas, refried beans, and bread pudding for dessert. That night, the organization promoted roasting marshmallows and chocolate s'mores around a bonfire. The next morning, the breakfast buffet featured, in the following order, bagels, cut fruit including pineapple, granola, breakfast cereal, and sugared yogurt before getting to the low-carb eggs and bacon.

Imagine this: a high-carb, high-fat emphasis throughout the weekend for a population of people with type 1 diabetes! It pained me to listen to the challenges and misery of people's lives in the sessions and then watch my new friends queue up and navigate the food choices. The conference conveners weren't being evil; they had simply succumbed to the fallacy of normalcy.

There's a movement away from emphasizing normal eating on the part of some mainstream experts, at least in terms of offering options. For example, at the 2019 TCOYD conference in San Diego, although Dr. Stephen Ponder demonstrated the use of CGM technology with the example of a cheeseburger with onion rings, he also covered surfing safer dietary waters, including a low-carb option.

The Language of Diabetes

The fallacy of normalcy is also promoted when the language is softened. We're not diabetics who suffer, instead we're people who just live with diabetes. We don't control the disease, we manage it; we don't test our blood, we check it.[14] The condition doesn't define us, and so on.

I understand this sentiment. To reiterate from an opening footnote, none of us wants to be defined by *what* we are rather than *who* we are. However, please consider the lesser of two evils and don't soften the language when you think of yourself. Sugarcoating isn't good for us, literally or figuratively. We do *suffer*. If we don't *control* diabetes, it will control us. We need to *test* our blood sugar via CGM or glucometer continuously, an ongoing test that spells life or death. Softening the language and sugarcoating, intended to make diabetic life more palatable and normal, ironically makes it tougher.

Diabetes is a serious disease state much like alcoholism. A recovering alcoholic at a twelve-step AA meeting doesn't hesitate to say, "Hi, I'm Bill, and I'm an alcoholic." Calling it out is part of acknowledging its seriousness. Why should our situation be any different?

Who would you rather be? An acknowledged person with diabetes thinking to yourself, *Hi, I'm Bill, and I'm a diabetic*, and eating an abnormally restricted diet to safely maintain healthy blood sugars using the minimum of medication possible—an approach that leads to glycemic stability, daily peace of mind, and better health? Or a person who happens to be living with diabetes—a person who, thanks to the miracle of drugs and devices, can and should eat pretty much like everyone else? Even though doing so may lead to diabetes distress, devastating complications, and possibly an early death?

I believe most people with diabetes would follow the first option *if they understood and knew about it*. Back in the day, I didn't think there was a choice. You might be in the same boat.

If you can see yourself as a person who lives in an abnormal disease state, and if you can accept simplifying and getting back to basics—even if that includes what a nondiabetic person might view as dietary deprivation—you're on the road to "I can do it!" You'll significantly improve your expectations and motivation. You'll be well on your way to positive change.

Questions for Your Care Providers

- *What should be the role of foods such as sugar, desserts, fast food, and sushi in my diet?*

- *Are there foods I should never eat?*

- *How do you feel about "cheat meals" and occasional desserts that may contain table sugar and high-fructose corn syrup?*

- *Other than carbohydrates, what other factors influence my blood sugars?*

The idea here is to assess your care providers' biases and understanding of factors affecting blood sugar other than carbs. Are their views nuanced to go beyond just how to cover carbs with medication? Are they aware of the forty-one factors other than insulin that influence blood sugar? Do they mention forbidden foods or dietary restrictions? (I hope so.)

- A question for you: *What tangible steps can you take to improve your first-level belief that, if you put forth the effort, you can improve your management of diabetes?*

Further Reading

BOOKS

- Alexander, Devin. *You Can Have It! More Than 125 Decadent Diabetes-Friendly Recipes.* Alexandria, VA: American Diabetes Association, 2018. (Tasty recipes. But see if you can combine meals with sides and a dessert and come in under 250 carb grams for a day.)

- Hill, Lewis Webb, and Rena S. Eckman. *The Starvation Treatment of Diabetes.* Boston: W. M. Leonard, 1916. (I'm not trying to depress you. But this little book gives perspective to deprivation. So we can't eat normally? We shouldn't eat sugar, desserts, fast food, and sushi? Big deal. In the old days, those with diabetes were dietarily deprived, sometimes to the point of starvation.)

- Jacoby, Richard P., and Raquel Baldelomar. *Sugar Crush: How to Reduce Inflammation, Reverse Nerve Damage, and Reclaim Good Health.* New York: Harper Wave, 2016.

- Lustig, Robert H. *Fat Chance: Beating the Odds against Sugar, Processed Food, Obesity, and Disease.* New York: Plume, 2012.

OTHER RESOURCES

- Dr. Jody Stanislaw's TEDx Talk "Sugar Is Not a Treat": TED.com/talks/jody_stanislaw_sugar_is_not_a_treat/transcript?language=en

CHAPTER 4

MORE ON THE MENTAL PART: FRAMEWORKS FOR SUCCESS

Acknowledging that our metabolism isn't normal, that we can't eat like other people, and that it's difficult—if not impossible—to successfully "cover" normal eating by relying on medication is just a starting point. The next steps are to eat, exercise, and otherwise live your life so you can maintain healthy blood sugars and achieve physiological homeostasis, or come as close to it as possible.

Homeostasis is important. It means achieving balanced metabolic stability and good numbers through healthy living rather than by relying on medication, including insulin. For example, an overweight person with T2D who has significant insulin resistance may normalize blood sugars each day by taking metformin and injecting 100 units of insulin; they may reduce blood pressure using 40 milligrams of an angiotensin-converting enzyme (ACE) and lower "bad" LDL cholesterol by taking 80 milligrams of atorvastatin. But they're not close to physiological balance, they're still storing fat, and their health is worsening. Healthy diabetic eating and exercise to safely maintain good blood sugars using a minimum of medication are essential for this person.* Ditto for someone with T1D who, because of an unhealthy diet and lack of exercise, must pump or inject 60 insulin units a day rather than a healthier 25 units.

A healthy homeostatic balance contributes to weight loss (if needed) and to maintaining a healthy weight primarily because less insulin is needed. Insulin is the fat-storage hormone. As Gary Taubes writes:

> Insulin works to deposit calories as fat and to inhibit the use of that fat for fuel. Dietary carbohydrates are required to allow this fat storage to occur. Since glucose is the primary stimulator of insulin secretion, the more carbohydrates consumed—or the more refined the carbohydrates—the greater the insulin secretion, and thus the greater the accumulation of fat.[1]

As insulin levels rise from poor diet choices, people get fatter.[2] (Ask any physician. They'll tell you their diabetic patients gain weight when insulin or a medication that increases insulin

---

* *But they and all others with diabetes should not change their diet or medications without first consulting their care provider.* This is particularly true for everyone who uses insulin or a blood sugar–lowering pill such as a sulfonylurea (glipizide, glimepiride, or glyburide). Other medications, such as for blood pressure, may also need to be adjusted or eliminated as weight falls.

secretion is prescribed.) It's also a physiological fact that most overweight and obese people lose weight when their insulin levels fall.[3]

So it's important to establish and then maintain lower insulin levels. This is true whether the insulin is pumped, injected with a pen, or secreted by pancreatic beta cells. I realize that insulin created in the body is not technically "medication." However, moving forward, I group it as such when writing about the need to minimize medication. We need to maintain healthy insulin levels regardless of where the hormone comes from.

The focus on dieting in the next two sections may seem inapplicable if you're height-weight proportionate. Please read on anyway. It's good information. Besides, these sections segue into a perspective that very much pertains to you and everyone else with diabetes.

The Chicken or the Egg?

What comes first? Intentional weight loss through "dieting" that leads to the need for less medication, including insulin? Or eating a diet that minimizes medication that leads to weight loss, but as a by-product, not as a purpose? I opt for the latter.

Weight loss by itself lowers insulin resistance and insulin levels and improves health. Traditionally, going with the first option, an overweight person with diabetes will "go on a diet." Pounds come off, medication levels fall, and health improves, but the fix is usually temporary for reasons I soon discuss.

The alternative is to instead focus on lifelong, healthy eating that safely lowers blood sugars using a minimum of medication (again, including insulin from all sources as "medication"). Weight loss in this scenario then becomes a *by-product of healthy living*, not the purpose of going on a diet. For a person with diabetes who doesn't need to lose weight, this alternative simply leads to stable weight maintenance and much better health.

I've been down both roads. I was diagnosed with type 1 diabetes in 1968. Twelve years ago, although my A1cs fell below the ADA's standard of 7.0 for good control, I was in hell, with my blood sugar bounding up and down all day long. What's more, I had become a "double diabetic"—obese with insulin resistance and cardiovascular disease. I tried a commercial diet program twice and flunked both times. Then I began eating low-carb, high-fat meals based on the philosophy of Dr. Richard Bernstein. A year later, I was forty pounds lighter and had cut my daily insulin load by 50 percent. My A1cs fell comfortably into a normal range—not for a person with diabetes but for a person in general.

My time in range, the period when blood sugar is between 70 and 180 mg/dL, has remained comfortably around 95 percent, with A1cs in the mid-5s to low 6s. For the past decade, my weight has varied, give or take, by only ten pounds. I wasn't dieting to lose weight; I was simply trying to better manage my blood sugar. Weight loss just happened, as did my reduced need for insulin and other medications.

It's Not Just Splitting Hairs

It might seem like splitting hairs. Does it matter if we "go on a diet" to lose weight to improve blood sugars *or* maintain healthy blood sugars with minimum medication so that weight loss occurs as a by-product, not a purpose? Well, the answer is "yes." The order does matter.

Dieting to lose weight and then hanging on with grim

determination to any weight loss to keep diabetes at bay is an abstraction compared to focusing on maintaining healthy blood sugar. The former is just about losing fat and somehow keeping it off. The latter speaks directly to diabetes itself as a permanent part of your life.

Also, you could lose twenty pounds by dieting and still have unhealthy blood sugar levels because of chaotic eating. Sure, over time, average insulin levels fall and the weight comes off. However, that may come with high-glycemic excursions caused by a given diet's "permission" for a weekly holiday or special treat days, a dynamic that soon contributes to the diet's failure. Any weight loss becomes temporary. The dieting cycle begins anew or the person just gives up.

A twenty-pound weight loss through dieting might also be inadequate. What if a forty-pound weight loss is needed to significantly improve insulin resistance and metabolic syndrome markers? You lose twenty pounds, but you still fail. Twenty pounds was hard enough! Plus, "going on a diet" to lose forty pounds is an aberration. No one eats like that forever! And the time required to lose forty pounds feels like forever.

There is also the self-defeating psychology of dieting to consider. When was the last time you went on a diet to lose weight without thinking of it as temporary? "Going on" a diet sets up the implicit expectation that you're going on something you'll eventually get off. Indeed, many diet programs reinforce this expectation with a maintenance phase that few can maintain.

On the other hand, a focus on healthy eating that safely maintains healthy blood sugars using a minimum of medication is not a temporary aberration. It's something we *must always do*, whether overweight or not, as part of everyday life because *we are and will always have diabetes.* And, in time, if needed, weight loss happens for most people.

A digression here: Despite claims to the contrary, although the condition can be reversed, type 2 diabetes can't be cured through weight loss. As with a sober alcoholic who will always be alcoholic, a person diagnosed with diabetes will stay that way. Even in remission, the condition simmers in the background. For those who once carried too many pounds, it lies in weight. (Pun intended!)

Moving on, even if you start the traditional route by going on a diet to lose weight, you're still okay if safely maintaining healthy blood sugars with as little (if any) medication as possible *becomes the new purpose.* Put another way, normalizing blood sugar (or as close to it as safely possible) relates directly to your permanent medical condition, as opposed to reducing the fat hanging around your belly. Doing the former addresses a cause rather than a symptom.

The balance of this chapter puts to rest the concept of "going on a diet" and replaces this thinking with a perspective that supports living a successful diabetes life.

The Futility of Going on a Diet

To reiterate from Chapter 2, most people with type 2 diabetes could throw away their medication if they lost enough weight. The doctor says to lose weight. But just how are you supposed to do this?

You might have a few sessions with a nutritionist who knows little about diet and diabetes drug interactions, or you might try a standard MyPlate or Mediterranean Diet. Either way, you go on a diet and start consuming "plenty of fruits and whole grains." Maybe you join a gym, but exercising doesn't help with weight loss, and the fruits and whole grains elevate your blood sugar just like the french fries of old. Any lost weight gets found again, and blood sugar levels remain unacceptable.

But you go on another diet anyway because you're not a quitter. In desperation, you might join millions of others and sign up for a diet program such as Weight Watchers, Jenny Craig, Medifast, and Nutrisystem. Between do-it-yourself dieting and a weight-loss program (or two or three), you find yourself back to the aforementioned insanity of doing the same thing repeatedly, expecting different results. Your first-level expectancy—the belief that your best efforts will lead to weight loss and better glycemic control—suffers. Yo-yo dieting may become a way of life, or you might just say "Screw it!" and give up.

Commercial weight-loss companies make a living off people with diabetes. That's not their fault. It's up to us to make sense of the futility of going on a diet. For example, does it make sense to go through formal stages of a weight-loss program eating packaged foodstuffs sold by the diet companies, and then somehow succeed after these supports are taken away? Or sign on for a diet that reintroduces or adds more to foods that were once unacceptable?

Many weight-loss programs have stages and use the concept of phasing back once-forbidden foods. Typical of this approach is the Atkins diet with its four stages: induction, ongoing weight loss, premaintenance, and maintenance—with varying amounts of allowable carbs at each stage. Atkins will also sell you a variety of low-carb foods and treats. But they're often only made to appear this way because of the company's use of the concept of net carbs, which are grams of total carbs minus nondigestible grams from dietary fiber. (I return to this topic in a future chapter. Accounting for net carbs is not as straightforward as it seems.)

Weight Watchers (now rebranded as WW) uses a point system for foods. It also has four stages: Honeymoon, The Thrill Is Gone, Renewed Resolve, and Lifestyle Change. More dietary points are allowed once you've hit Lifestyle Change and are on maintenance mode. The organization also sells a variety of supposedly healthy foods that include high-carb, two-point treats such as Mint Cookie Crunch Bars and Chocolate Caramel Mini Bars. (I loved those things, pounding them down all day long when I failed the diet repeatedly years ago.)

In short, staging the eating process and bringing back once-forbidden foods or larger amounts of food is self-defeating. For starters, we can't live forever on packaged processed foods sold by these companies. Then there's our old enemy, the slippery slope. *Okay, I finally reached the stage where I can eat potatoes, or more of them. They sure taste good. Think I'll take more medication and eat just a few more because I'm enjoying a special occasion.* And—*bam!*—I'm sliding back to bad eating and then on to another diet a few months down the road—probably a different one because the last one didn't work.

Commercial diet programs can also be expensive. In 2017, Americans poured over $68 billion into diet companies.[4] A year of Jenny Craig in the United States can cost over seven thousand dollars![5] There's also the relativity issue. For example, you might temporarily lose weight on a high-fat, low-carb diet or a low-fat, high-carb diet. However, this didn't happen because the diet was high or low in fat per se. It occurred because significantly reducing one of the three macronutrients of fat, protein, and carbohydrate meant you ingested significantly less food *relative* to the amounts of macronutrients you had been eating. You lost weight, not because of dietary magic, but because you took in fewer calories.

Dennis Pollock makes this point with the ice-cream diet. Of course, no one should live on ice cream alone, but if you ate only small amounts of it at each meal, morning, noon, and night, even though ice cream is full of carbs, you'd still need less insulin, store less fat, and lose more weight relative to your previous standard American diet.[6] All moot points. Unless you're one of the very few, the weight won't stay off.

Just how unsuccessful is dieting? A 95 percent failure rate is widely cited on the internet and in academic and popular literature, although this number is purportedly derived from a single 1959 obesity study.[7] A study of fourteen of television's *The Biggest Loser* participants found that half weighed more than when they had appeared on the show six years prior. The other half, successful "maintainers" according to the authors, still regained significant weight and remained obese, despite maintaining an average weight loss of 24.9 percent. A single participant lost all the weight and kept it off. This lone success out of fourteen leaves a 93.8 percent failure rate for a diet program that involved thirty weeks of intense, supervised exercise, training, nutritional counseling, and national attention.[8]

A single six-year follow-up of fourteen reality-show participants certainly doesn't validate a 95 percent failure rate, but it's sure a good example of the futility of dieting. The truth is that no one really knows how bad the failure rate is. You might as well throw darts at a Ouija board. And the scientific research hasn't helped; studies tend to be short-term, compare one dietary extreme to another, are based on unreliable self-reports, or all these things. For example, we may learn that a high-fat, low-carb diet leads to more weight loss than a low-fat, high-carb diet, but the trial lasted only six weeks or six months and was based solely on the potentially unreliable food diaries kept by subjects.

Here's a concluding remark from a published review of twelve weight-loss studies that shows the problem with diet research: "Weight changes were small; however, and weight regain was common. There were few similarities between the included studies; consequently, an overall interpretation of the results was difficult to make."[9] Another example of futility is seen in an analysis of again twelve weight-loss studies involving 6,754 diabetic participants. The authors flat-out conclude that weight loss for most overweight or obese diabetics might not be a realistic primary treatment strategy for improving blood sugars.[10]

At first glance, the results looked promising from Look AHEAD (Action for Health in Diabetes), the longest, most comprehensive weight-loss trial ever conducted involving people with diabetes.[11] The study, an eight-year randomized clinical trial of over five thousand overweight or obese people with type 2 diabetes, sought to determine whether a diet intervention reduced cardiovascular events between two study groups: a treatment group that received lifestyle counseling and dietary restrictions, and a control group.

The good news was that the treatment group lost significantly more weight after the first year and, although half of this weight was regained, it still showed a 4 percent loss at its conclusion. A third of the treatment group even maintained a moderate to large weight loss after eight years. The bad news: The study required intensive, ongoing individual and group lifestyle counseling and special diet foods, which are both deal breakers for most of us. And to add insult to injury, the special diet didn't reduce heart attacks.

The longest weight-loss study ever conducted, the National

Weight Control Registry (NWCR), began in 1994. Rather than embarking on a randomized controlled study seeking to confirm a hypothesis, researchers Drs. Rena Wing and James O. Hill simply began collecting information on dieters who keep the weight off. To join the registry, you need to be at least eighteen years old, have lost thirty pounds, and have kept the weight off for a year. Eighty-seven percent of NWCR participants maintain at least a 10 percent weight loss ten years after losing weight.[12] Over five thousand people are registered for the study.

It's an elegant idea: cut to the chase, publish what works, and give people the chance to replicate it. Alas, the researchers didn't find the One True Answer. Generally, they found a wide variety of dietary habits among those who successfully lost weight and kept it off. Specifically, four characteristics of successful dieters stood out; they:[13]

1. Cut calories to lose weight. In other words, they ate less. A wide variety of diets were used.

2. Self-monitored, weighing themselves regularly.

3. Exercised regularly, both during dieting and maintenance stages. Doing so didn't help as much with weight loss, but it contributed significantly to weight maintenance.

4. Ate a less-varied diet and limited binge eating during special occasions.

The following are the conclusions from the NWCR findings as they relate to diabetes.

Cut calories. Although fat is calorically denser than carbs and proteins, even a high-fat, low-carb diet still leads to fewer calories. (Recall my earlier point about the impact of significantly limiting one of the three macronutrients, in this case, carbohydrates?) In this example, you still can't overeat fat or protein. Although the carb-insulin-fat–storage pathway is the number-one weight gainer, fat, protein, or both also affect blood sugar and insulin levels and can metabolize into weight gain through alternative metabolic pathways.

Calorie reduction will also occur because you no longer permit yourself to eat heavy or inappropriate meals, since you understand that covering excessive or inappropriate carbs with medication is not the answer.

Self-monitor. NWCR participants regularly tracked their weight using the bathroom scale. People with diabetes who are overweight or obese should do this as well, but self-monitoring should also include regular blood sugar checks with a glucometer or CGM.

Exercise regularly. The NWCR participants demonstrated the power of exercise to maintain weight loss, but not to lose it. Regular exercise, ideally every day, is also a crucial part of keeping blood sugar low and within the target range. Chapter 7 addresses how to make the right amount of exercise doable and bearable in everyday life. A key takeaway is that you don't have to like exercise. The good news is that it doesn't take a lot to be healthy, and it becomes bearable if treated as a rote activity of daily life, like brushing your teeth or taking a shower.

Eat a less-varied diet and avoid bingeing. Eating a less-varied diet comes with the territory. As is covered in the next chapter, eating a low-carb, high-fat diet as most of us should do, or the plant-based high-carb, low-fat exception, makes food less varied. That's just the way it is. We can't have our cake and eat it too. But we still have it pretty good compared to the past. Thrice-boiled cruciferous vegetables with whiskey-spiked coffee used to be what many people with diabetes ate until they died of starvation.[14]

Adapting and Applying a Twelve-Step Perspective

So, you get it. You understand the fallacy of normalcy. You realize that relying on medication to cover carbohydrates from normal eating isn't the answer. That dieting by itself is futile. That weight loss—to the extent that it's needed and it occurs— and weight maintenance should be viewed as a by-product of healthy, permanent eating (and exercising) to safely maintain healthy blood sugars, using a minimum of medication, not the purpose of going on a diet. You've figured out and are ready to practice a healthy daily diet and exercise program. You'll monitor your weight regularly using the bathroom scale and your blood sugar with a glucometer or CGM.

All good, but just to a point. Necessary, but still insufficient. There's still something missing: a perspective that holds understanding and practice together each day, without which we run the risk of joining the myriad ranks of those who try and fail. I close this chapter with a paradigm familiar to many, and one that I have found personally helpful.

You might consider adapting and applying an Alcoholics Anonymous (AA) twelve-step perspective to your everyday management of diabetes. Now, before you incredulously fall out of your chair, please consider that poorly controlled diabetes and alcoholism have much in common. Both:

- Cause chaos and disruption in everyday life, leading to distress

- Negatively affect family members in a variety of ways, including ongoing social and emotional impacts

- Contribute to "policing behavior" by concerned family members

- Involve an unhealthy consumption of dietary substances that target pleasure centers in the brain

- May lead to guilt, manipulation, and acting out associated with this consumption

- Are expensive

- Contribute to poor health, are progressive, and, unless arrested, cause or contribute significantly to death

Twelve-step recovering alcoholics strive to be in the present. For this day, and this day alone, they seek to be sober. The next day, the process repeats, and so on for the rest of their days. A person with diabetes can apply the same perspective. *Today, I will eat healthy food and only healthy food. I will engage in at least a modicum of healthy exercise. Tomorrow, the same. One day at a time.*

Doing otherwise means falling off the wagon. It'll be tough in the beginning. You may have to fake it until you make it. But it's worthwhile because the stakes are high. Know that you at least have the choice. You don't have to agree with the "sushi hack" mentioned in Chapter 3 or with endocrinologist Dr. Jeremy Pettus's recommendation of "f**k it" times, when you eat whatever you want, from his presentations at recent TCOYD conferences. I respectfully disagree with these views. You can too.

Fortunately, there's more to a twelve-step philosophy than just abstinence. There's a spiritual component that is "an active relationship with a power greater than yourself that gives your life meaning and purpose."[15] Otherwise, without spirituality, without daily purpose, if we focus just on food—particularly on what we can't eat—we may become a "dry drunk," smacking our lips and lashing out at people.

The spiritual piece might be your relationship with God or even God as you understand Him (or Her!). If you want to keep God out of it, you might focus on your relationship with *whomever or whatever you love more than yourself.* A *what* rather than a *who* you love more than yourself might consist of an egalitarian commitment to a local cause or an organization. Personally, my wife, Patty, and my two children, David and Kevin, are people I love more than myself. (Back in my college days, because of my diabetes, a campus physician told me to never father children. I'm glad he was wrong.)

Support from others on the same path is also key. Alcoholics Anonymous meetings are widely available for this purpose, and a sponsor is assigned to each member. People with diabetes have less structured opportunities to interact, though a variety of possibilities are available through local health care or diabetes organizations. However, it can be tough to connect in these venues with those specifically trying to safely maintain healthy blood sugars using a minimum of medication. You might consider recruiting a diabetic friend for support who has read this book or is otherwise in tune with its concepts. This person wouldn't be like an AA sponsor but would be more like a person on the same journey, such as my T1D friend Alice, with whom I walk and talk.

Applying a twelve-step perspective to day-to-day living with diabetes holds much promise. For example, AA reports that 36 percent of its members have been sober for more than ten years; Overeaters Anonymous claims a 54 percent success rate. In the academic literature, sobriety success rates range from 5 to 8 percent after one year, and up to 67 percent for regular AA participants after sixteen years.[16]

How well applying this perspective works in a diabetes life lies somewhere between these extremes, but I submit to you that it carries a greater potential for success in terms of staying off the glycemic roller coaster and avoiding diabetic complications than do the alternatives of gritting your teeth each day to keep weight off—or, for those who are height-weight proportionate, blithely covering whatever you eat with medication because you've not experienced negative consequences (at least not yet).

There is a diabetes twelve-step group called the Recovery Group (http://www.therecoverygroup.org/special/diabetes.html). However, this group is overly focused on the harm of compulsive overeating, not on safely managing blood sugar using a minimum of medication. Their approach is all about food, and their target audience is overweight or obese people with T2D. A related option of joining a diet-focused twelve-step program like Overeaters Anonymous to lose weight, improve blood sugar, and call it good has the same problems.

A twelve-step perspective in diabetes management doesn't exclude those who are height-weight proportionate because it's not about weight loss. It's about safely managing blood sugar one day at a time, emphasizing diet and exercise using a minimum of medication rather than dropping pounds. To reiterate, this approach keeps in mind that weight loss, to the extent it is needed or occurs, should be viewed as a by-product of healthy diabetic living, not the purpose of a diet.

If you apply a twelve-step perspective to managing your diabetes, you'll practice six steps, not twelve like a recovering alcoholic, and you won't attend meetings, conduct a moral inventory, or make amends for past behavior, but the overarching focus on purposefully living in the present is the same:

1. Define a healthy daily diet and exercise program (covered in the next three chapters).

2. Be in the present. Live one day at a time.

3. Commit to a daily, disciplined practice of a healthy diet and exercise program. Put another way, abstain from unhealthy eating and exercise habits each and every day.

4. Define and live each day with an overriding spirituality and purpose.

5. Seek out reciprocal support from at least one or more fellow travelers who share your blood sugar goals and management needs.

6. Work closely with your care provider to stage minimizing medication needs and, of course, for all other health matters as well.

To conclude, be sure to work with your care provider to stage medication needs based on your daily diet and exercise program. *You must have this conversation before you begin a new pattern of eating and exercising.* For most, especially those who are overweight or obese and experiencing insulin resistance and metabolic syndrome, the process could take several months. Diabetes medication amounts and types will change based on a new eating pattern and as weight drops. Other medications may also need adjusting such as those for cholesterol or blood pressure.

Regardless of your weight, it's important to keep in mind that over time, out-of-control blood sugar changes the equilibrium point at which the body tolerates lower blood sugar. For example, if your average blood sugar runs very high, say, above 250 mg/dl, you could feel hypoglycemia with an otherwise normal blood sugar of 100 mg/dl. This is another reason to work closely with your care provider before changing how you eat and exercise.

The next two chapters cover nutrition, the next most important part of the hierarchy of diabetes care.

Ginger Vieira Weighs In on the Mental Part

Mental health in diabetes is about resilience. We're all human. And a diabetes diagnosis doesn't change that. Everyone in life has challenges, and diabetes is one of our challenges. I've lived with type 1 diabetes for twenty-one years. For the past fifteen years, I've met and worked with hundreds of others with type 1, type 1.5, and type 2 diabetes, and they all have something in common: They're human, too.

Diabetes doesn't just add stress to our lives; our lives add stress to diabetes. This means that managing your mental health needs to include room for imperfections, for stepping back a little sometimes, for making "mistakes," for

continued

learning from "mistakes," and for improving your self-care gradually over years and years. *Over years and years*, rather than trying to become the "perfect" diabetic overnight.

This means that *resilience* is actually the most critical tool in your diabetes toolbox. Resilience is your ability to wake up every single morning and face your diabetes management duties again and again, regardless of how things went the day before.

Resilience is also about *protecting* your mental health because diabetes management comes with so much pressure, so many rules, so many warnings, so many tasks, and so many tests.

Some days, your *best effort* may look awesome on that glucose meter or in your choices around food, medications, and exercise. On other days, your *best effort* may look a little less awesome. Giving yourself room to be human—rather than beating yourself up for imperfections—is what will help you wake up the next day with renewed resilience and energy to face diabetes all over again.

What you know about your diabetes today versus what you'll know ten years from now will be vastly different if you view every high or low blood sugar as merely an opportunity to learn something new. Dust off. Try again. Rinse and repeat.

Resilience.

Diabetes management consumes a tremendous amount of our mental energy—even if you're thriving and have healthy routines in place. When something else in life happens—like a divorce, the death of a loved one, a sick family member, changes in your career, going to college, breaking up with your boyfriend or girlfriend, and so on—these things inevitably take energy away from diabetes management. And sometimes that's okay. (Of course, as long as you're still doing the basics to keep yourself out of the hospital!)

Your mental health is also affected by the rules and beliefs you develop around your physical health. It's been all-too-well established that diabetes and eating disorders go painfully hand-in-hand—that's because diabetes inevitably creates such a hyper-focus on food—and an endless list of lectures about what we can and cannot, should and should not, eat. "Bad" foods versus "good" foods. Beliefs that we are "bad diabetics" for eating "bad" foods.

In my experience, most people with diabetes thrive when they protect their own mental health by giving themselves grace and flexibility and by finding out what works for them versus trying to adhere to what works for someone else.

While Chad and I may disagree on how people with diabetes "should" eat, our goal is the same: for you to thrive in life with diabetes.

But you are truly in charge of what happens next, and that actually comes down to determining what works best for you. Many readers may try a twelve-step perspective as Chad suggests to nutrition and thrive, while others may struggle immensely. This isn't because you're a failure or you lack discipline. It's because there is no "one size fits all" to diabetes management or *life* in general.

Me? I thrive with the freedom to choose. There are no

continued

rules—there are simply decisions I make, and because I get to be in charge, I am empowered to make lots of really healthy choices, with room for less-than-perfect choices.

What works for you? What helps you feel empowered by your relationship with food and diabetes? What helps you feel empowered by your relationship with exercise? With your blood sugars? With your health care team?

The secret to thriving both mentally and physically isn't about copying what someone else is doing, but rather taking the same steps they took in simply experimenting and determining what works best *for you*.

You picked up this book because you're looking to improve your life with diabetes, and there's no doubt that this book will guide you in that process! If you find the twelve-step perspective approach to food to be too restrictive, that doesn't mean you're a failure.

As Bruce Lee once said, "Use only that which works and take it from any place you can find it."[17]

Use the ideas in this book to create your own sustainable approach to thriving with diabetes—thriving both physically and mentally, because you can't have one without the other.

And most of all: Give yourself some room to be imperfect. Don't beat yourself up when you trip and fall. Get up. Dust yourself off. Take a deep breath. And try again, perhaps with a few tweaks in your approach next time.

Experiment and develop an approach that you can successfully sustain. A strict low-carb approach might work for years and years, and then something in your life or your beliefs and knowledge about nutrition might change, and so your approach changes, too.

Chad may not know this, but I ate strictly low carb *for years*—and it worked well for me during that time of my life. But today, the strictness of how I used to eat doesn't feel like a healthy fit for me, mentally or physically. And guess what? My A1c isn't higher. My insulin needs are *lower*. And actually, I weigh *less*. It's not because there's one secret fix to diabetes; it's because my life and my beliefs about what balanced nutrition looks like for me at this time in my life have changed.

It's about *you* and the details in *your* life—the details that make up who you are, the challenges you face, the strengths you possess, and the things that bring you joy. Chad has researched and describes approaches that work well for him, both mentally and physically.

And now it's your turn.

Don't forget to carry a handful of resilience with you wherever you go.

* * *

Ginger Vieira has lived with type 1 diabetes and celiac disease since 1999 and fibromyalgia since 2014. She is the author of four books: *Pregnancy with Type 1 Diabetes*, *Dealing with Diabetes Burnout*, *Emotional Eating with Diabetes*, and *Your Diabetes Science Experiment*. Her background includes a BS in professional writing and certifications in coaching, personal training, and yoga. Ginger

continued

creates content regularly for diabetes websites, including *DiabetesMine*, *Healthline*, Omnipod, *Diabetes Strong*, Diathrive, DiabetesSisters, YouTube, Instagram, and many more. She helped develop the diabetes coaching program for InquisitHealth and speaks regularly at diabetes conferences, camps, and organizations. Once upon a time, Ginger set fourteen records in drug-free powerlifting, but just as she let go of intense nutrition rules, she stepped away from intense exercise, too. Today, Ginger lives in Vermont, where you'll find her writing, jumping rope, running around with her daughters, or walking with her handsome fella, Karl, and their dog, Petey.

Questions for Your Care Providers

- *Do I have insulin resistance? If so, to what extent?* Your physician may speak with you about blood pressure, cholesterol, blood sugar, current medication levels, and possibly other markers for insulin resistance and metabolic syndrome. Those with type 1 diabetes should keep in mind that they, too, can have insulin resistance.

- *What factors are important to improve insulin sensitivity?*

- For those with T2D: *If I enter into a healthy eating and exercise program, over time, what medications can be eliminated? In what order and timetable might we stage their elimination or otherwise modify their use?* If you've had long-standing type 2 diabetes, you may be taking several diabetes medications as well as insulin. Your care provider should be qualified to work through a hypothetical progression with you and must be involved, particularly if you are using insulin or blood sugar-lowering medications.

- For those with T1D: *If I enter into a healthy eating and exercise program, over time in what order and by what timetable might we stage a reduction in medications, especially insulin?*

Further Reading

- Fitzgerald, Matt. *Diet Cults: The Surprising Fallacy at the Core of Nutrition Fads and a Guide to Healthy Eating for the Rest of Us.* New York: Pegasus Books, 2014. (A well-written and researched look at the futility of going on a diet.)

- Pollock, Dennis. *You Can Achieve Normal Blood Sugar: Discover the Surprising Results from over 100 Blood Sugar Tests.* Eugene, OR: Harvest House, 2019. (Pollock does a great job of connecting food with blood sugar.)

- Wilson, William G. ("Bill W."). *Alcoholics Anonymous: The Story of How Many Thousands of Men and Women Have Recovered from Alcoholism.* New York: Alcoholics Anonymous World Services, 1939. (Of course, AA's "Big Book" isn't about diabetes, but it includes insights into successful daily coping with a chronic disease.)

- Munn, Jeffrey. *Staying Sober without God: The Practical 12 Steps to Long-Term Recovery from Alcoholism and Addiction.* Self-published, 2019. (For those who wish to leave religion out of it, this book also gives insights into daily coping with disease.)

CHAPTER 5

BALANCING MACRONUTRIENTS AND THE RULES

Nutrition is involved in all parts of the hierarchy of diabetes care for a good reason. As a renowned diabetes expert, endocrinologist Dr. Irl Hirsch, once said, "Food is the key!!!"[1] It's too bad the topic is so confusing.

Nutrition opinions ripple out from thousands of self-help books, often with acrimony and finger-pointing. Witness *The Low Carb Myth* (Ari Whitten and Wade Smith, 2015) and *The Low-Carb Fraud* (T. Colin Campbell and Howard Jacobson, 2014) on one side of the fence, and *The Big Fat Surprise* (Nina Teicholz, 2014) on the other. Some titles suggest we're being fooled in general: *The Diet Delusion* (Gary Taubes, 2008) and *Diet Cults* (Matt Fitzgerald, 2014). Eggs and bacon smile or frown up at us from book and magazine covers. For most writers, the attitude is "If I'm right—and I am—then you must be wrong."

It's the plant-based, high-carbohydrate, low-fat people versus the low-carb, high-fat people. It's all so confusing and tiring, and some of the advice is questionable. For example, the author of *The Starch Solution* believes that blood sugar in a toxic range between 150 and 300 mg/dL is good control. He still relies on urine sugar data with his patients, a standard of care outdated by more than thirty-five years.[2] Of course, in sniping at this fellow, I'm guilty of the partisanship that typifies the literature. (Do you see the problem?)

In surveying the popular literature, the fable of the blind men and the elephant comes to mind. You know the story: A group of blind men encounters an elephant, a creature they had never experienced. Each man grabs a different part of the pachyderm—one man a tusk, another the tail, and so on. Each concludes the nature of the whole elephant from this very limited experience, and of course, they all disagree.

This dynamic can be seen in attributions for insulin resistance. Dr. Neal Barnard believes fat in the form of intramyocellular lipid is the cause. According to Dr. Barnard, too much dietary fat clogs up the cells, making it more difficult for insulin to let in glucose, thereby increasing insulin resistance and raising blood sugar.[3] Dr. Jason Fung has a different view: Too much high blood sugar and hyperinsulinemia from the high-carb, high-fat standard American diet (SAD) stuffs cells with too much glucose, thereby increasing insulin resistance and pushing circulating glucose away to storage as glycogen and fat.[4] Both authors subsequently justify their diet recommendations based on their respective positions: Dr. Barnard's high-carb and low-fat solution to steer fat away from clogging up cells; Dr. Fung's low-carb and high-fat approach to reduce glucose from carbs being forced into overloaded cells.

Countering views among diet experts have occurred because they can. Our bodies are an adaptive miracle with alternative metabolic pathways that have evolved to flourish ideally in homeostasis on a wide variety of macronutrients. People, in general, can be healthy eating a wide variety of foods. But the food must be real, not from a package, box, or fast-food restaurant, and there must be enough protein (but not too much, unless you're building muscle or are highly active).

Still, we are not "people in general." *The situation for us is different.* Most of us need to restrict carbohydrates to be healthy, though there is an exception soon to be discussed.

The Goals of Diabetic Nutrition

To reiterate, the primary goal of diabetic eating, together with exercise, is to safely maintain healthy blood sugars using the minimum of medication possible. Controlling blood sugar means not just improving an average as measured by A1c but also keeping it at a healthy time in range.

A second goal is to adequately nourish the body with the calories, vitamins, minerals, and fiber necessary to stabilize weight and maintain good health. I focus on the former in this chapter because improving blood sugar average and time in range using a minimum of medication should be our most important dietary goals.

Blood Sugar Average and Time in Range

A healthy blood sugar range typically falls between 83 and 99 mg/dL over twenty-four hours, although blood sugar can peak up to 120 mg/dL in a nondiabetic person one to two hours after eating, depending on the type and amount of carbohydrate consumed. A healthy A1c of 4.9 percent falls into this range as an average two-month blood sugar of 94 mg/dL; a prediabetic A1c of 5.9 percent means an unhealthy average blood sugar of 123 mg/dL. The ADA sets an A1c below 7.0 percent as the definition of good control, an average blood sugar of 154 mg/dL. The American Association of Clinical Endocrinologists sets the bar lower at 6.5 percent, with an average blood sugar of 140 mg/dL.[5] The ADA has decreed a diagnosis of diabetes at above 6.5 A1c. Note: Using an A1c value to diagnose diabetes isn't like turning on or off a light switch. You may not officially have diabetes at 6.4, but you're still in trouble.

Lowering average blood sugar reduces or eliminates long-term complications. For example, one T2D study found *each* 1 percent reduction in A1c was associated with a reduction of risk of 21 percent for any end-point-related diabetes complication, and 37 percent for microvascular complications.[6] The early 1990s Diabetes Control and Complications Trial (DCCT) famously found that lower blood sugars led to a significant reduction in complications for those with T1D. The results were so convincing that the study was suspended a year early.

It's not clear to what extent lower average blood sugar or the reduced insulin loads that accompanied this lower blood sugar contributed to fewer complications in these studies. It's tricky because a chronically high insulin level (hyperinsulinemia) by itself can be toxic.[7] However, the fact that benefits are associated with lower blood sugar is indisputable. Consequently, the simple answer for most of us is to go as low as safely possible. According to Dr. Bernstein, we're entitled to—and should strive for—the same blood sugars as those without diabetes.[8] But there's a catch.

The rub lies in safety. Another study, the Action to Control Cardiovascular Risk in Diabetes (ACCORD), was also suspended early (in 2008), but not because of a favorable result. The subjects in the intensive treatment group died at a significantly higher rate than those in the control group. It's not understood why this occurred, but the study used higher-risk older subjects with a mean age of sixty-two, with over one-third having already had a cardiovascular event. It's conceivable that tighter control in the intensive treatment group led to fatal cardiovascular events caused by hypoglycemia.[9] An implication from these findings is that average blood sugar targets should be personalized with the active assistance of a care provider so that they are both low *and* safe.

Improving time in range also contributes to better diabetes outcomes.[10] This metric deals with the percentage of time a person with diabetes spends between an ideal of 70 mg/dL and 180 mg/dL. A person with diabetes can achieve the ADA's A1c 7.0 cutoff for tight control but with a daily time in range of only 50 percent.[11] This seems a low bar. With the right diet and reduced medication, you can achieve a much better percentage (I'm in the 90s). *But this is difficult, if not impossible, to do with the standard American diet and a high medication load.* Be sure to talk with your care provider about this.

Now begins the most complex part of this book. Please bear with me as I work my way through it. I begin by telling a story. I experienced a miracle when I read Dr. Bernstein's book twelve years ago and started eating a low-carb, high-fat diet. I lost copious weight as a by-product of healthy eating using less medication; my blood sugar averages and time in range normalized, and my cholesterol and blood pressure numbers improved significantly. Hypoglycemia decreased. My success continues to this day. For example, a recent angiogram confirmed that my coronary plaque has stabilized. I became, and continue to be, a devotee of lower-carb eating.

I wanted to learn more about this low-carb miracle, plus Dr. Bernstein's excellent book piqued my interest in nutrition. So I started to read both academic and popular literature. Eight years later, I finally started to write this book. It took this long to sort out my ideas. What I thought was a straightforward proposition turned into "fighting a land war in Asia." The complexity of interfaces involving nutrition and physiology as influenced by genetics, physical activity, and psychology boggled my mind. The countering views of all the experts were overwhelming. I've made some sense of things, but discussion of nutrition and diabetes by anyone, by its nature, will always be incomplete.

The bottom line? *Most* (but not all!) of those with diabetes need to eat fewer carbs to improve, even normalize, blood sugar in terms of average and time in range, particularly when blood sugar-lowering medication is in the picture. Otherwise, trying to cover high-carb eating with medication, especially insulin, leads to unhealthy glycemic unpredictability and difficulty in safely sustaining healthy blood sugar. Dr. Bernstein observes that big inputs of carbs and medication create big mistakes, while small inputs make small mistakes. He then states:

If you can't accurately predict your blood sugar levels, then you can't accurately predict your needs for insulin or oral blood sugar-lowering agents. If the kinds of foods you're eating give you consistently unpredictable blood sugar levels, then it will be impossible to normalize blood sugars.[12]

But as you'll see in the next section, there is a high-carb, plant-based exception for some. You'll find that the other macronutrients—fat and protein—are also part of maintaining healthy blood sugars.

Finding a Healthy Macronutrient Balance

Before considering the macronutrient components of a healthy diet, it's important to cross one option off the list—the Western diet, also known as the standard American diet (SAD). This eating pattern emphasizes high-carb *and* high-fat eating together, a deadly duo that has sickened humans across the globe.

Consider breakfast in the United States of eggs, hash browns, buttered toast, and bacon with a glass of orange juice followed by lunch of a fast-food cheeseburger, fries, and a milkshake. Dinner that night might be more fast food or mounds of mashed potatoes, sausage gravy, and fried chicken, followed by blueberry pie with whipped cream. It's not just the large number of calories that's problematic. It's also the combination of high fat *and* high carbs consumed simultaneously during that day and all the days that follow.

Another aspect of the deadly duo concerns the nature of the carbohydrates consumed—highly refined and highly glycemic. The story might have a happier ending if the carbs were instead from lower-glycemic, non-starchy vegetables such as broccoli, cabbage, or cauliflower, but they're not. White foods—potatoes, bread, pasta, rice, flour, and refined sugar—are the most important players here and become truly deadly when fat joins the party. For example, by adding Alfredo sauce to pasta or breading to a chicken-fried steak.

Deadly-duo fast foods such as pizza, cheeseburgers, and burritos make up one-third of American meals.[13] Foods eaten quickly and conveniently at home also enter the picture: Hamburger Helper, mac and cheese, Pop-Tarts, and sugary breakfast cereals. Add snacks between meals, such as candy bars, potato chips, soda, and cookies. All these high-carb, high-fat, processed foods, eaten day after day, week after week, year after year, soon have a body yelling, "Help!"

This steady rain leads to insulin resistance, metabolic syndrome, weight gain, and long-term complications associated with elevated blood glucose. Blood glucose levels stay high because, as previously noted, fat slows down carbohydrate and protein metabolism by increasing insulin resistance, delaying gastric emptying, or both. This extends after-meal blood sugar levels far longer than is healthy. In one study, a sample of pizza eaters maintained a rise in blood sugar up to *nine hours* past that of a control group.[14]

A healthy metabolism can tolerate moderate portions of white rice, pasta, and white bread, even at every meal, but not if that metabolism is also simultaneously and regularly hit with large amounts of any kind of fat and the protein that usually comes with it and that person is also sedentary. People with diabetes should consider a different macronutrient balance as outlined in Figure 5.1.

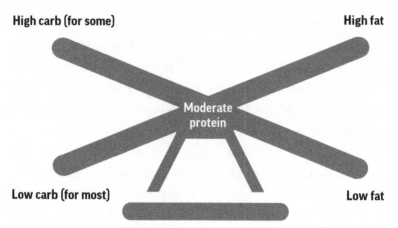

High carb (for some)

High fat

Moderate
protein

Low carb (for most)

Low fat

Figure 5.1. The macronutrient teeter-totter for people with diabetes.

Of the three macronutrients—carbohydrates, fats, and protein—dietary carbs and fats should balance one another. It's like a teeter-totter. *If one of these two macronutrients is high, then the other must be low.* The low-carb, high-fat plank works for all people with diabetes. However, an exception can be made that opens the high-carb, low-fat plank to some who eat a plant-based diet.

Protein sits moderately in the middle for all. Unless you're trying to build muscle or engage in regular and vigorous exercise, you don't need a lot of it. An otherwise healthy, sedentary sixty-seven-year-old, six-foot-tall, two-hundred-pound male eating low-carb at 125 grams per day requires only 12.1 ounces of protein daily. The same person with the addition of heavy exercise only needs 13.6 ounces per day.[15] Another reason to eat protein conservatively is that it raises blood sugar significantly more so than does dietary fat.[16]

LOW-CARB, HIGH-FAT WORKS FOR ALL

The low-carb, high-fat plank on the teeter-totter helps manage diabetes effectively and safely using a minimum of medication. It works for all of us. And it's not unhealthy.

A case in point is the story of Vilhjalmur Stefansson. This early twentieth-century Arctic explorer flourished for four years on a very low-carb, high-fat diet while living with the native Inuit.[17] Upon his return to the United States, Stefansson ate only meat during a tightly controlled one-year diet study. At the request of the researchers, he initially ate a very high-protein diet that consisted of lean meat with little fat. He became sick, only restoring his health after being allowed high-fat meats.[18]

In his later writing, Stefansson describes the extreme fat hunger of "rabbit starvation," the plight of forest Indians during tough times who got sick from high-protein, low-fat subsistence on rabbits, the leanest meat source.[19] The bottom line: We need healthy dietary fat, and it's not bad for us.

There are two variations on the low-carb, high-fat plank of the teeter-totter. The first is ketogenic. Ketones are produced in the liver from burning fat, which becomes an alternative fuel on a very low-carb diet when insufficient glucose is available for energy from other macronutrients, especially carbohydrates. A metabolism can become wholly ketone-adapted as opposed to carbohydrate-adapted.[20]

It's widely held among mainstream researchers and writers that glucose, not ketones, is the body's preferred energy source. Others disagree.[21] What can be said for sure is that ketone production, ketosis, and a keto-adapted metabolism are normal, as evidenced by the example of the Arctic Inuit and Vilhjalmur Stefansson and by the personal experience of diabetes expert Dr. Richard Bernstein and his patients. (Dr. Bernstein, who has

T1D himself, safely normalizes blood sugars with a minimum of medication on a daily ketogenic diet that includes only 6 grams of carbohydrate at breakfast, 12 at lunch, and 12 at dinner.)

You don't need to restrict carbs as much as Dr. Bernstein's diet to become keto-adapted and stay that way. The more you weigh, the more carb grams you can eat and stay in ketosis. A keto-adapted metabolism can be maintained with as many as 50 to 70 carb grams daily, depending on body weight.

A second, more moderate lower-carb approach, one that I now practice, keeps the body just above ketosis at about 100 to 125 carb grams consumed per day, again depending on body weight. My body still primarily burns glucose from carbohydrates for energy, but the insulin needed at this level is still low relative to the standard American diet, and fat storage is discouraged.

Don't fear ketosis or ketone bodies. Particularly, don't confuse potentially deadly diabetic ketoacidosis (DKA) with the normal dietary ketosis as experienced by the native Arctic Inuit and Dr. Bernstein, or ketone production during the night as the body taps fat stores.

Don't go ketogenic if you have kidney problems, are pregnant, or are insulin-dependent and poorly controlled. Above all, *be sure to consult with your care provider* before making the switch. Once started, I recommend that you not abruptly drop carbs in favor of fat. Make the transition slowly. You otherwise run the risk of developing "keto flu," becoming constipated and just generally feeling miserable.

You can get good advice on ketogenic eating from a couple of the books listed at the end of the chapter: *Dr. Bernstein's Diabetes* and *The Ketogenic Diet for Type 1 Diabetes* authored by en Davis and Keith Runyan. The latter book is good for th type 2 diabetes as well.

And don't be afraid of eating fat.

DIETARY FAT IS HEALTHY

Since the late 1970s, dietary fat, especially saturated fat, has been demonized as the guilty party by US government policy. The primary reason was the diet-heart hypothesis promoted by researcher Ancel Keys.[22] This hypothesis supported the idea that cholesterol causes cardiovascular disease in part because arterial plaque is composed of cholesterol. Saturated fat causes a rise in cholesterol, particularly "bad" LDL cholesterol. Therefore, eating saturated fat must cause cardiovascular disease. Right?

Nutritionists subsequently told us to avoid eating fat because it "clogs" arteries, as though the fat in steak leaps from the knife and fork to a landing zone in our cardiovascular system. Food marketers jumped on the bandwagon and began cranking out "lite" and "low-fat" foods and promoting processed vegetable oils for frying and baking, all supposedly healthier because they had less effect on LDL levels. Carbs replaced fat. People ate these foods instead of eggs and bacon and switched to margarine containing damaging trans fats rather than butter composed of saturated fat (remember SnackWell cookies?). Over the past fifty years in an increasingly sedentary society, this switch contributed to weight gain, cardiovascular disease, and diabetes.*

Recent studies refute the diet-heart hypothesis. Eating saturated fat is not associated with all-cause mortality, cardiovascular

---

* This is one point of view. Another espoused by author T. Colin Campbell and other high-carb, plant-based advocates is that Western society never truly did go "low-fat." Fat intake was reduced but not enough to make a difference. Consequently, we were left with the deadly duo of high-carb, relatively high-fat eating that leads to obesity, metabolic syndrome, and diabetes.

disease, coronary heart disease, ischemic stroke, or T2D, although trans fats are.[23] (For a comprehensive review of eighteen other studies saying that saturated fat isn't the problem, go to nutritioncoalition.us/saturated-fats-do-they-cause-heart-disease.) Except in rare cases of familial hypercholesterolemia, though saturated fats do increase LDL cholesterol levels, this does not, *by itself,* cause cardiovascular disease or predict the likelihood of having a cardiovascular event.[24] Usually, other negative factors are in play along with high LDL when a heart attack or stroke occurs. Many of them are associated with metabolic syndrome and T2D: high blood pressure, arterial inflammation, low "good" HDL cholesterol, high triglycerides, insulin resistance, and being overweight or obese.

Genetic risk factors that get little attention from care providers also contribute significantly to cardiovascular disease. An inherited elevated lipoprotein(a) level, or Lp(a), *triples* the chance of a heart attack independently of other risk factors.[25] Additionally, fifty other genetic risk variants or markers have been confirmed for coronary artery disease, most of which are uncorrelated with the conventional risk factors listed in the preceding paragraph.[26]

Given this foregoing information, it's not surprising that you might as well flip a coin to determine the value of having a low LDL cholesterol number. Half of all hospital admissions for cardiovascular events record "healthy" low LDL levels below 100 mg/dL.[27] The reality is that dietary cholesterol is essential to good health. And, in fact, most cholesterol—over 80 percent—is produced in our liver, *not from the food we eat.*

So don't be afraid of eating fat in general, saturated fat specifically, or cholesterol. But do fear trans fats, which are created through hydrogenation—the heating of liquid vegetable oils in the presence of hydrogen gas and a catalyst.

The US Food and Drug Administration (FDA) banned trans fats effective June 18, 2018, although foods manufactured before this date could still be distributed until 2020 and, for some foods, until 2021. Also, if food has fewer than 0.5 grams of trans fat per serving, it can read zero trans fats on the label.[28] Trans fats were banned because they indisputably contribute to cardiovascular disease. Check the ingredients. Stay away from any food that lists partially hydrogenated oil or hydrogenated oil.

THE HIGH-CARB, LOW-FAT EXCEPTION FOR SOME

To reiterate, eating a high-carb diet doesn't seem to make sense for a person with diabetes. Our pancreatic beta cells can't handle high carb loads, producing too little or no insulin in the case of type 1 diabetes, and too much, and later sometimes too little, in the case of type 2 diabetes accompanied by metabolic syndrome and insulin resistance.

However, the recommended diet of Dr. George King of the Joslin Clinic, described as the plant-based, high-fiber rural Asian diet (RAD), might be just the ticket for a person with T2D who may pack a few extra pounds, is physically active, and still has functioning pancreatic beta cells.[29] A case for the diet can also be made for a height-weight-proportionate person with T1D who has exceptionally well-managed diabetes. In other words, the diet might work for those of us who are not obese and who do not need multiple diabetes drugs to manage our disease.

The macronutrient proportions of Dr. King's diet—70 percent complex carbs, 15 percent fat, and 15 percent protein—are the same as the diet of the South American Tsimané people, who have the lowest reported levels of coronary artery disease ever recorded.[30] Hundreds of millions of rural Asians have prospered eating this diet. Dr. T. Colin Campbell's well-known China Study reports the same benefits for a comparable population.[31]

Another example of successful plant-based, high-carb, very low-fat eating is covered by Dr. Cyrus Khambatta and Robby Barbaro, who both have type 1 diabetes.[32] The diet advocated by these authors works because it reduces dietary fat to below 30 grams daily, thereby reducing insulin resistance associated with eating fat and making insulin significantly more efficient. Thankfully so—because both of the authors consume up to *700 carb grams per day* using fewer than 30 units of insulin each. Up to 19 units of mealtime boluses are part of the daily picture for each fellow. That's a carb-to-mealtime insulin ratio of 37 to 1! (My hat's off to them. I'm at a much less efficient ratio of 11 to 1.)

It's a strange world where these authors, the Tsimané, and rural Asians are as healthy as Dr. Bernstein, the blubber-eating Inuit, and the milk-, meat-, and blood-consuming Maasai nomads of Kenya, who, in 1962, like the Tsimané, had very little cardiovascular disease and, at the time, the lowest blood-cholesterol levels ever measured.[33]

The above examples underscore the miracle of alternative metabolic pathways and demonstrate that some of us have options. However, for the reasons to follow, most of us are still better off eating a lower-carb or even a ketogenic diet.

WHY THE LOW-CARB PLANK IS STILL BEST (FOR MOST OF US)

Overweight or obese people with diabetes don't do well on high-carb diets. A study published in the *New England Journal of Medicine* reports that severely obese subjects with a high prevalence of diabetes or metabolic syndrome lost more weight after six months on a low-carb diet than on a calorie- and fat-restricted high-carb diet.[34] This finding is consistent across studies.[35]

Dr. Walter Willett of the Harvard Medical School, one of the most respected nutrition experts on the planet, notes that overweight people do worse on high-carb diets than do lean people. After citing research showing unhealthy changes in HDL cholesterol and triglycerides levels among these individuals, he states, "Put more plainly, a low-fat, high-carbohydrate diet may be among the worst eating strategies for someone who is overweight and not physically active."[36]

In making this point, Dr. Willett doesn't dispute the benefits of plant-based complex carbohydrates. The question is, what's a better plank on the teeter-totter if a person with diabetes and metabolic syndrome carries an extra fifty pounds? The high-carb plank that tends to increase insulin levels (even if from eating healthy plants) or a lower-carb or ketogenic diet that minimizes fat storage via the carbohydrate-insulin pathway? It makes more sense to opt for the latter.

For those who bolus insulin, the potential for hypoglycemia with high-carb eating and insulin dosing is also an issue. I acknowledge that dietary fat increases insulin resistance, making insulin less efficient. Consequently, it's possible for a highly active person who avoids dietary fat to have a highly efficient carb-to-mealtime insulin ratio, such as Dr. Khambatta and Mr. Barbaro's 37 to 1. However, I'd be uncomfortable with the average of more than six units of fast-acting insulin they require for each meal, not counting occasional correction boluses. Peace of mind comes from small mealtime boluses that are possible with ketogenic or lower-carb eating. For me, that's four or fewer units per meal with the occasional small correction bolus.

Smaller boluses are also supported by Dr. Bernstein's previously discussed rule: big inputs make big mistakes; small inputs make small mistakes. No glycemic roller-coaster rides!

Another problem is the emphasis placed on a vegetarian, often vegan, diet in high-carb, low-fat diet books. Most of us don't want to eat this way, and it's not necessary to be healthy. We have, after all, evolved to become omnivores!

And still another problem with many plant-based authors is their ideological hammering, much like the proselytizing you might expect from a religious missionary. An example is their use of the term "nutrient-dense" when referring to plant foods, as though red meat isn't. Red meat is healthy. It's more nutrient-dense than soybeans, legumes, or peanut butter. It's a source of B vitamins, L-carnitine, iron, conjugated linoleic acid, carnosine, zinc, selenium, and phosphorus. And vegans may need supplementation with vitamin B12 because, as acknowledged by Dr. Khambatta and Mr. Barbaro in their book, this essential vitamin doesn't come from plants.

There is also their unequivocal, relentless, unnuanced support for the failed diet-heart hypothesis of Ancel Keys. Finally, in reading on both sides of the fence, it has seemed to me that some "planters" spend excessive effort discrediting the other side. Slamming another point of view doesn't make you right. (I realize that some irony is happening here.)

And can insulin-dependent people with diabetes possibly eat massive carbs and avoid glycemic disaster? I planned a dietary experiment to explore this issue. Fortunately, Ginger

Vieira, with T1D herself, beat me to it.[†] I believe I would have had the same problems Ms. Vieira had.

Of course, you might disagree with me. If so, research confirms that you're still vastly better off with the high-carb, plant-based diet of a rural Asian, a Tsimané, or Dr. Khambatta and Mr. Barbaro than you are with the deadly duo SAD diet of a typical American.[37]

Next Steps

You've picked your plank on the teeter-totter. Next, the rules. No one likes rules, but that's the situation. (Feel free to call them "guidelines" if that sounds better.) As twelve-step thinkers, we need to eat healthily one day at a time, bound by the same rules that apply to recovering alcoholics, who not only can't imbibe but also need to stay away from bars and taverns. These rules are based on what the different diets promoted by the gurus *have in common* and on the list of foods that were once forbidden for all of us but that the fallacy of normalcy now permits.

The experts universally agree that healthy food and diets are low in added sugar, eliminate refined carbs, avoid processed vegetable oils high in omega-6 fats, eschew trans fats, are high in vegetables and fiber, and focus on the quality of food rather than just counting calories.[38] The experts universally support eating food that is cooked at home in the kitchen from individual ingredients, rather than processed boxed or canned options that need only a microwave or stove for reheating. The experts

---

†   For a well-balanced and detailed description of her experience with Dr. Khambatta and Mr. Barbaro's diet, go to diabetesstrong.com/my-high-carb-low-fat-experiment-with-type-1-diabetes.

oppose most fast food. The tricky part of the agreement among them, other than the proportions of macronutrients, concerns the nature of veggies.

Experts on the low-carb high-fat plank recommend against eating starchy vegetables such as beets, corn, carrots, and potatoes. Pasta, rice, and white bread are also off-limits. High-carb, low-fat advocates allow these foods but qualify their support by recommending that they be made with whole grains such as oats and bran rather than processed grains. The experts universally agree on the benefit of eating cruciferous vegetables such as kale, cauliflower, broccoli, brussels sprouts, bok choy, cabbage, collard greens, rutabaga, parsnips, and turnips, and other above-ground veggies such as green beans, peas, asparagus, and spinach.

Fruit is also a point of contention. They all agree that fruit juice is verboten. You might as well put vitamin C in soda pop. But whole fruit is a different matter. It's loaded with fructose (bad) but includes healthy micronutrients, as well as dietary fiber that slows down blood sugar spikes (good). If you're going low-carb, you should still eat whole fruit sparingly, including tomatoes and tomato sauce. But everyone can eat avocados!

Next comes the list of traditionally forbidden foods. This list is based on the first point on which all diet experts agree: the need to eliminate added sugar and refined carbs. In the old days, the ADA included such a list with its traditional exchange diets before it switched to advocating for dietary diversity. The traditional forbidden foods are powdered, brown, or granulated sugars, as well as corn sugar or syrup, honey, molasses, maple syrup, chips, jams and jellies, cake, cookies, candy, frosting, granola bars, ice cream, pie, pastries, sweet rolls, donuts, sugared soda, and sugared cereals.

The website where I found this list recommends that people with diabetes "carefully use these foods" or otherwise talk with a dietitian and eat only the foods on the list they say are okay.[39] Good grief! Nothing is okay with eating poison. Regardless of which plank you're on, skip the talk with the dietitian, mentally affix a skull and crossbones to these foods, and just say no.

To conclude, the six rules of healthy diabetic eating boil down to the following.

1. *Don't fear eating fat or cholesterol, and saturated fat in particular.* Eat as few trans fats as possible—ideally none. Use olive or coconut oil rather than processed vegetable oils.

2. *If you pick a low-carb plank (as most should), eat sparingly (if at all) whole fruit and starchy veggies,* such as corn, carrots, beets, and potatoes. Instead, consume cruciferous vegetables such as kale, cauliflower, broccoli, brussels sprouts, bok choy, cabbage, collard greens, rutabaga, parsnips, and turnips. Add green beans, peas, asparagus, and spinach. Any vegetable grown above ground can be added to the list.

3. *For the minority who can succeed with the high-carb plank, this doesn't mean eating rice, pasta, or bread made with refined grains.* Instead, eat small amounts of whole-grain versions of these foods and otherwise get your carbs predominately from the "good" vegetables listed above and from beans and lentils. Think of the high-carb plank as a high-fiber, plant-based, whole-food diet. This means a minimum of rice, pasta, potatoes, and bread, even if they're made with the good whole-grain stuff.

4. *No drinking fruit juice or eating traditionally forbidden foods:* powdered, brown, or granulated sugars, as well as corn

sugar or syrup, honey, molasses, maple syrup, chips, jams and jellies, cake, cookies, candy, frosting, granola bars, ice cream, pie, pastries, sweet rolls, donuts, sugared soda, and sugared cereals.

Fruit juice and sugary junk food should only be consumed in a low-blood-sugar emergency. If you have a choice, you're still much better off using dextrose tabs or eating Smarties or Skittles to treat lows. These choices are faster and more reliable.

5. *Eat the vegetables, fish, meat, poultry, and eggs found on the outer edges of the grocery store* rather than the processed, packaged foods on the shelves in its interior. Ideally, the protein comes from wild-caught, pasture-raised, or free-range sources. No fast food. However, choose a salad if you must.

6. *Eat a less-varied diet; don't binge, and eat this way every day,* regardless of whatever holiday or special occasion is occurring. (This advice comes from National Weight Control Registry [NWCR] findings.) Finally, you will find that though calories do matter, counting them isn't as important as is their nature. The next chapter continues this point.

Questions for Your Care Providers

- *What are your views of dietary fat and cholesterol?* Does your care provider understand that dietary fat and cholesterol are no longer the bad guys? For example, that eggs are okay to eat? That a fat-based diet by itself isn't going to give you a heart attack? Do they understand why it may be difficult, if not impossible, for you to maintain healthy blood sugars using a minimum of medication while also eating the carbohydrate load of an otherwise healthy standard MyPlate or Mediterranean Diet?

- For those considering a ketogenic diet: *What are the challenges, dangers, or both of such a diet?*

- *Will you consider ordering an NMR LipoProfile test for me?* Traditionally, simple LDL, HDL, and total cholesterol tests are ordered by your care provider. From these numbers, cardiovascular risk is estimated. LDL is "bad" because it purportedly contributes to forming arterial plaque, so a low number is good. (That's why many people take a statin to drive down this number.) HDL is "good" because it transports LDL away, so the higher the better. Of course, as noted in the chapter, it's not that simple. LDL levels, unless extremely high, are not generally predictive of a cardiovascular event.

  But there's more to the story. The nature of cholesterol particles also matters. The NMR LipoProfile panel takes a closer look at this issue. For example, it assesses whether LDL particles are of pattern B, the dense, arterial-burrowing, inflammation-causing, plaque-forming type, or pattern A, the large fluffy type that safely bounces off the arterial walls. A healthy diet and exercise contribute to the homeostasis that reduces insulin resistance, and it also has the beneficial effect of changing the LDL-particle pattern type from the bad B to the good A. This transformation is a marker of improved health. Consequently, it might be helpful to check your current particle status and, through future testing, the progress you make after changing how you eat and exercise.

- *Will you consider ordering an Lp(a) test for me?* This simple, inexpensive blood test lets you know if you have inherited elevated Lp(a) cholesterol, a factor that significantly predicts a heart attack. Statins don't affect Lp(a). Some trade book authors and bloggers argue that large doses of over-the-counter niacin successfully treat the condition. But niacin has potential problems of its own. At the very least, an elevated Lp(a) may encourage you to work harder on those nutrition and exercise factors you can control to safely maintain healthy blood sugars using as little medication as safely possible. Be sure to discuss these issues with your care provider.

- *How might I improve my blood sugar time in range?*

- For those who are insulin-dependent: *How do I account for protein and fat when bolusing insulin for meals?* Mealtime bolusing that goes beyond carbs is a complex, important topic worthy of discussion with your care provider. Dr. Maria Muccioli does a great job of covering the complexities in a February 2022 *Diabetes Daily* online column recommended in the next section.

Further Reading

BOOKS

The following books cover both planks on the macronutrient teeter-totter. They are representative of the dietary differences and recommendations passionately and articulately expressed (and some that aren't) in thousands of books, articles, and blogs.

- Bernstein, Richard K. *The Diabetes Diet.* New York: Little, Brown Spark, 2005.

- Bowden, Jonny. *Living Low Carb: Controlled-Carbohydrate Eating for Long-Term Weight Loss.* New York: Sterling, 2013.

- Bowden, Jonny, and Stephen Sinatra. *The Great Cholesterol Myth.* Beverly, MA: Fair Winds Press, 2012.

- Cole, Will. *Ketotarian: The (Mostly) Plant-Based Plan to Burn Fat, Boost Your Energy, Crush Your Cravings, and Calm Inflammation.* New York: Avery, 2018. (This is a good book to read if you're seeking a plant-based, low-carb diet option.)

- Davis, Ellen, and Keith Runyan. *The Ketogenic Diet for Type 1 Diabetes: Reduce Your HbA1c and Avoid Diabetic Complications.* Cheyenne, WY: Gutsy Badger, 2017. (This book is good for those with T2D as well.)

- Khambatta, Cyrus, and Robby Barbaro. *Mastering Diabetes: The Revolutionary Method to Reverse Insulin Resistance Permanently in Type 1, Type 1.5, Type 2, Prediabetes, and Gestational Diabetes.* New York: Avery, 2020.

- King, George L. *Reverse Your Diabetes in 12 Weeks: The Scientifically Proven Program to Avoid, Control, and Turn Around Your Diabetes.* New York: Workman, 2016.

- Stone, Gene, ed. *Forks over Knives: The Plant-Based Way to Health.* New York: Experiment, 2011.

- Taubes, Gary. *Why We Get Fat and What to Do about It.* New York: Anchor Books, 2010. (This is a shortened, more readable version of Taubes's *Good Calories, Bad Calories: Fats, Carbs, and the Controversial Science of Diet and Health* [New York: Anchor Books, 2008].)

- Vieira, Ginger. *Your Diabetes Science Experiment: Live Your Life with Diabetes Instead of Letting Diabetes Live Your Life.* Burlington, VT: Living in Progress, 2010.

- Volek, Jeff S., and Stephen D. Phinney. *The Art and Science of Low Carbohydrate Living: An Expert Guide to Making the Life-Saving Benefits of Carbohydrate Restriction Sustainable and Enjoyable.* Miami, FL: Beyond Obesity, 2011.

OTHER RESOURCES

- Jonathan Bailor's TEDx Talk, "Can Superman End Diabetes?": youtube.com/watch?v=JUF5yF9LZCg.

- *Healthline*: healthline.com. This is a good source of nutrition information, particularly if the column is authored by Kris Gunnars. (Another online nutrition columnist to follow is Chris Kresser.)

- *Fed Up*. Directed by Stephanie Soechtig. Atlas Films, 2014. This documentary is about ninety minutes long and is available on Netflix and from other regular outlets.

- *Forks over Knives.* Directed by Lee Fulkerson. Monica Beach Media, 2011. This is a documentary about a plant-based, high-carb, very low-fat diet (see the book of the same name listed above). The documentary is available on a variety of streaming video providers (see forksoverknives .com/the-film).

- Muccioli, Maria. "How to Calculate Bolus Insulin Dosing for Protein." *Diabetes Daily*, February 12, 2022. https://www.diabetesdaily.com/learn-about -diabetes/treatment/insulin-101/how-to-use-insulin/ how-to-calculate-bolus-insulin-dosing-for-protein.

- *Why Are We Fat?* Directed by Mark McNeill and Will Sergeant. Razor Films, 2016. This is a three-part, three-hour series available on a variety of streaming video providers such as Amazon Prime and Netflix.

CHAPTER 6

MAKING SENSE OF NUTRITION, CALORIES, FIBER, AND HEALTHY EATING

This chapter moves through the topics of calories and dietary fiber and then concludes with a framework for building a healthy diet.

The term *diet* used in this section refers to a plan for eating, not "dieting" for weight loss. We all eat a diet, but we should never go on one!

Making Sense of Calories

A calorie is a unit of energy derived from food. We take in calories, and our bodies burn this energy as needed for activities ranging from breathing and sleeping to sitting in front of the

TV and running a marathon. The concept of calories hasn't been around all that long. The US Department of Agriculture's first research director, Wilbur Atwater, introduced the concept in a government pamphlet in 1894 that listed the protein, fat, and carbohydrate calories of common foods.

Atwater determined that 4 calories of energy are derived from 1 gram of protein or carbohydrate, and 9 calories from 1 gram of fat.[1] It then became possible to calculate, in Atwater's words, the total food energy value required by an American male laborer or a sedentary female office worker. For example, Atwater recommended the laborer consume more than 3,000 calories per day, with 52 percent of this energy total from carbs, 33 percent from fat, and 15 percent from protein.

Weight loss soon became connected to the need to reduce dietary calories. A pound could be lost by eating 3,500 fewer calories than the body needed for energy, by expending 3,500 calories of energy greater than the calories consumed, or by a combination of the two. Since the early 1940s, the Metropolitan Life Insurance company has famously maintained height-weight charts depicting, by height, the range from ideal weight to obesity. Since then, care providers and their patients have used this type of information to set weight-loss goals. Using caloric-deficit thinking based on a chart and whether the "diet" cut five hundred calories daily, losing thirty pounds to hit an ideal weight could be achieved in thirty weeks.

The process of creating a caloric deficit to lose weight through "dieting" proportionately ramped up through the decades with the fattening of the developed world. For example, a recent CDC study found that about half of all adult Americans now go on diets, even though counting calories expressly to lose weight fails 95 percent of the time and is futile for the reasons covered in Chapter 4.[2]

Calorie counting is a troubled construct. The energy-in, energy-out model is simplistic. It doesn't address the quality or nature of food, just the energy it generates. For example, a five-hundred-calorie serving of table sugar and one of broccoli has the same caloric value even though these foods affect the body including blood sugar very differently. Simply gaining or losing weight based on 3,500 calories per pound also runs smack-dab into the "set point" dilemma, whereby intricate metabolic physiology slows down weight loss at a certain point, no matter what.

For sure, the indigenous Inuit, Tsimané, and Maasai peoples and rural Asian farmworkers didn't count calories (or even care what they were) and maintained healthy weights with very little diabetes.

Diets on different planks of the diabetes macronutrient teeter-totter covered in the previous chapter also aren't based on calories. Dr. Bernstein tells people with diabetes that within his guidelines, "You can eat what you want and like to eat."[3] Dr. King states that the height-weight-proportionate among us "can eat as many calories as you want—provided you stay within the diet's nutritional guidelines."[4]

Along the same lines, Jonathan Bailor, in his excellent book *The Calorie Myth*, builds a compelling case in favor of the *quality* of food eaten, not the *quantity* as measured by calories.[5] High-quality calories promote satiety, are less likely to be stored as body fat, and are nutritionally dense.

In short, calorie counting is flawed. *What* you eat is as important, if not more so, as *how much* you eat, as measured by calories. Drs. Bernstein and King and Mr. Bailor generally agree. Indigenous people eating native diets without concern for calories do great. So, should we be concerned with calories at all? The answer, albeit qualified, is yes.

The Role of Calories

I propose using calories not for calculating an energy deficit to lose weight but as a starting point for determining the number of macronutrients, particularly carbs, needed to safely maintain healthy blood sugars using a minimum of medication. This use is temporary and just for planning purposes.

What should your caloric starting point be? There are myriad calorie calculators to help with this. For example, using the calculator available at healthline.com/nutrition/how-many-calories-per-day, I filled in the blanks—5'11", 170 pounds, active lifestyle—to determine that I require 2,697 calories daily.

Of course, it goes without saying (but I'll say it anyway) that your care providers need to be part of the decision process as well. They might recommend a weight-loss diet, meaning your daily caloric starting point minus the proverbial five hundred calories. I'm not a fan of doing this, since weight loss should be a by-product of healthy eating, not a purpose. However, you might still go down this road. No worries *if you realize this reduction is permanent*. It should be permanent for several reasons: first, because it's part of a necessary mindset; second, because we should never "go on a diet"; and last, because fewer calories are needed if you weigh less, something that invariably occurs if you need to lose weight and begin to eat healthily. Dr. Bernstein says this well:

> What you eat when you're losing weight will be essentially what you eat as you're maintaining your weight over the long term. . . . You'll start the diet, lose weight, and once your weight has leveled off at your target, you'll stay on the same essential regimen you followed while losing weight.[6]

After you figure out your total calories, the next step is to design a diet based on the proportion of carbs, protein, and fat calories needed depending on your plank on the teeter-totter. Table 6.1 depicts representative proportions.

Table 6.1. Macronutrient proportions for different diets

Diet	Carbohydrates	Protein	Fat
Low-carb, high-fat (ketogenic)	5–10%	15–25%	70–80%
Lower-carb, high-fat	20–25%	15–25%	55–65%
High-carb, low-fat (RAD diet)	70%	15%	15%

At 4 calories per gram for carbohydrate and protein, and 9 calories per gram for fat, a daily 2,000-calorie, lower-carbo-hydrate diet might have 125 carb grams (25 percent of total calories), 75 protein grams (15 percent of calories), and 133 fat grams (60 percent). To get to these numbers, we needed the starting point of 2,000 calories.

We're talking approximations. In this example, the starting proportions are based on 1,997 calories, not 2,000 calories. I'm also not going to plot a diet that has me *precisely* eating 125 grams of carbs a day. For me, it might be 120 one day, 130 on another. It's okay to be approximate with carbs, within the spirit of your plank on the nutritional teeter-totter, unless you're eat-ing a ketogenic diet and are on the ketosis boundary. In this case, as discussed earlier, you need to stay below the ketosis carb limit based on your body weight.

Macronutrient proportions can also vary depending on the person. For example, Table 6.1 holds at 15 percent of calories from protein across the board to emphasize that calories from protein should be constant and moderate regardless of the proportions of carbs and fat. However, you'll need more protein each day if you're more active, but not a lot. To reiterate from Chapter 5, a sedentary sixty-seven-year-old, six-foot-tall, two-hundred-pound male eating a low-carb diet of 125 grams per day requires only 12.1 ounces of protein daily. The same person with the addition of heavy exercise needs only 13.6 ounces per day.

Making Sense of Dietary Fiber

You also need adequate dietary fiber, that nondigestible carbohydrate found mostly in plant foods such as fruits, vegetables, legumes, whole grains, nuts, and seeds. The US Dietary Guidelines published by the USDA recommend the daily ingestion of 38 grams of fiber for men and 25 grams for women. Americans eat significantly less than those amounts—an average of 16.2 grams daily, according to one study.[7]

The benefits of fiber are many, extending far beyond improving bowel regularity. People who eat a lot of fiber are at significantly lower risk for developing coronary heart disease, stroke, hypertension, diabetes, obesity, and gastrointestinal diseases. They have lower blood pressure and cholesterol levels and—important for us—improved glycemic and insulin sensitivity.[8] Their trillions of gut bacteria necessary for health are also better off.

The classification of fiber is a complex subject. There are soluble and insoluble types. The former is the fiber that dissolves in liquid versus fiber that does not. There are also fermentable and resistant starch categories of fiber. There are subcategories; for example, viscous fiber is a subset of soluble fiber. Different types of fiber have different benefits. For instance, only the viscous fiber found in whole foods such as asparagus and brussels sprouts reduces food intake and contributes to weight loss.[9] We can cut through this complexity, since our goal is to safely maintain healthy blood sugars using a minimum of medication. Consequently, the specific upside of subtypes is less important than is fiber's overall benefit to lessen blood sugar spikes after meals.

Getting to 30 or more fiber grams per day is a no-brainer if you're part of the minority who can sit on the high-carb, very low-fat plank. This plank emphasizes whole plant-based foods that provide plenty of fiber of all types. Getting to a fiber goal on a ketogenic or a lower-carb, high-fat diet is a harder row to hoe. Speaking of garden rows, you can still get there by focusing on above-ground and cruciferous vegetables as much as possible. Berries such as raspberries and blueberries can be added to the list. Berries are surprisingly low-carb and full of fiber.

Supplementation can help. You could consider adding a fiber supplement such as psyllium husks. That's not a bad idea in general. Fiber supplementation with psyllium improves conventional markers of glycemic control in those with T2D beyond usual care.[10] With food, eating two avocados a day adds 26 grams of fiber with negligible carbs. (I know it seems oxymoronic to eat a "food supplement." However, it's still supplementation if, for health reasons, you eat something daily that you normally wouldn't.)

Fiber also enters the picture when calculating "net carbs"

derived by subtracting nondigestible grams of carbohydrate from fiber from those that are digestible. The idea of net carbs is widely viewed as an invention of food manufacturers to improve sales, particularly to low-carb dieters or people with diabetes. There isn't a legal definition; nor is there FDA regulation. The ADA does not have an official position on the subject.

Calculating net carb grams is easy to do with whole foods. Simply subtract the fiber from the total carbs. For example, there are 4 net carb grams in an avocado—17 carb grams minus 13 grams of fiber. It's trickier to do with processed foods because they contain sugar alcohols and possibly glycerin that have a minimal effect on blood sugar, and a wide variation exists among the experts on the best approach.* I conclude this section with ideas for making this calculation.

On the face of it, the concept of net carbs is attractive; it's an opportunity to benefit from "free calories" to splurge on specially modified candy and other goodies. For example, Figure 6.1 depicts a 23-carb-gram Atkins chocolate peanut bar shrunk down on the label to just *3* digestible net carbs. It looks good on the surface, but there are issues. For example, I'd have problems if I covered only 3 net carb grams of an Atkins bar with insulin. I know from experience that my blood sugar would rise unexpectedly and significantly.

---

* Sugar alcohols include mannitol, maltitol, maltitol syrup, lactitol, xylitol, erythritol, sorbitol, hydrogenated starch hydrolysates, and isomalt. Their calorie content ranges from 0 to 3 calories per gram compared to 4 calories per gram for sucrose or other sugars. Some affect blood sugar more than others; for example, maltitol significantly more so than erythritol. Sugar alcohols can cause significant gastric distress. Glycerin is an organic compound found in plants and is known more formally as glycerol. Common sources are vegetable oil and animal fat. Glycerin is also used in the food industry as a filler and thickening agent. Outside of food, it's used to make soap and is in some pharmaceutical and cosmetic products.

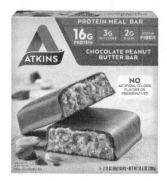

Nutrition Facts
Serving Size 1 Bar (60g)

Amount Per Serving

Calories 250	Fat Calories 130	
		% Daily Value
Total Fat 14g		22%
Saturated Fat 8g		40%
Trans Fat 0g		
Polyunsaturated Fat 1g		
Monounsaturated Fat 3g		
Cholesterol 5mg		2%
Sodium 250mg		10%
Potassium 210mg		6%
Total Carbohydrate 23g		8%
Dietary Fiber 12g		48%
Sugars 2g		
Glycerin 8g		
Protein 16g		20%
Vitamin A 0% • Vitamin C		0%
Calcium 6% • Iron		8%

Percent Daily Values are based on a 2,000 calorie diet. Your Daily Values may be higher or lower depending on your calorie needs.

	Calories:	2,000	2,500
Total Fat	Less than	65g	80g
Saturated Fat	Less than	20g	25g
Cholesterol	Less than	300mg	300mg
Sodium	Less than	2,400mg	2,400mg
Potassium		3,500mg	3,500mg
Total Carb		300g	375g
Dietary Fiber		25g	30g
Protein		50g	65g

Calories per gram: Fat 9 • Carbohydrates 4 • Protein 4

'Counting Net Carbs? Glycerin is naturally sourced from vegetables and gives our bars a soft texture. Glycerin and fiber should be subtracted from the total carbs since they minimally impact blood sugar.

TOTAL CARBS (23g) - FIBER (12g) - GLYCERIN (8g) =

3g ATKINS NET CARBS

No Maltitol

INGREDIENTS: PROTEIN BLEND (SOY PROTEIN ISOLATE, GELATIN, WHEY PROTEIN ISOLATE, WHEY PROTEIN CONCENTRATE), POLYDEXTROSE, PEANUTS, VEGETABLE GLYCERIN, PALM KERNEL AND PALM OIL, NATURAL FLAVOR, WATER, COCOA POWDER (PROCESSED WITH ALKALI), CELLULOSE POWDER, CONTAINS LESS THAN 2% OF: PEANUT OIL, BUTTERFAT, SOY LECITHIN, OLIVE OIL, MILK, SALT, GUAR GUM, SUCRALOSE.

CONTAINS MILK, SOY, PEANUTS.

Figure 6.1. Atkins Chocolate Peanut Butter Bar. (© 2020 Simply Good Foods USA, Inc. Atkins® and the Atkins logo are registered trademarks of Simply Good Foods USA, Inc. Use of any Atkins trademarks, logos, and product names does not imply endorsement.)

Dreamfields pasta is another example. The pasta was delicious, but its effect was no different for me and others than regular pasta. Although the company denied allegations of mislabeling, it paid $7.9 million to settle a class-action lawsuit around the issue.[11] Still another example concerned the Quest Peanut Butter Protein Bar. A diabetes support group found that, on average, an unexpected blood sugar increase of 50 mg/dL resulted from the product. The company graciously communicated with the group to search for answers, but satisfying ones weren't to be found.[12]

So, what makes sense when it comes to accounting for net carbs? The answer is that it depends. For those who bolus insulin for meals, you could follow Dr. Bernstein's advice and deduct half of the stated grams of fiber from the stated grams of carbohydrate for all foods to get a *general* idea of how the listed carbohydrate will affect your blood sugars and dose accordingly.[13] You could be more refined and subtract all the fiber, glycerin, erythritol, and half of all the other sugar alcohols.

For insulin users, the main thing is to err on the side of under-dosing, but not to the extreme that occurs when 23 carb grams become only 3. Whatever you do, don't overdose! Previously, I mentioned the problems with hyperglycemia from covering just 3 net carbs, but I'd also overdose if I bolused for all 23 grams of carbohydrate.

If you eat low-net-carb processed food, you might consider experimenting with the foods you eat regularly. For example, I regularly eat Mission Carb Balance tortillas, which are 6 net carb grams after subtracting 13 grams of fiber from 19 carb grams. But I don't bolus for 6 net grams. Instead, I bolus for half of the total carbs from the food, about 10 grams (rounding up), rather than for 6. Not wanting to underdose or overdose, I had to carefully experiment to get to this conclusion.

If you don't bolus for meals, you could disregard the whole net carb issue. Eat a healthy diet as defined. Stay away from pro-cessed goodies and candy that tout low net carbs. Net carbs just don't matter if you're already safely maintaining healthy blood sugars using a minimum of medication and following the six rules of healthy diabetic eating.

ding a Diet

What's left is to create and follow a diet based on your macronutrient numbers. Then, as you learn from your blood sugar readings and as you tweak while you eat, you'll know how and what to eat permanently.

A good starting place is to find a representative diet book, or books, that fit the plank you've chosen. For example, the Atkins diet book or Dr. Bernstein's recipe book listed at the end of this chapter includes classic low-carb, ketogenic recipes. A less restrictive lower-carb/high-fat plan can be constructed by tweaking ketogenic recipes to add a few healthier grams of carbohydrate.

The high-carb, very low-fat, plant-based plank can be accommodated using a Pritikin diet book (for example, see pritikin.com/14-day-menu.html).† You could also check out the high-carb, low-fat recipes from *Mastering Diabetes* or *Forks over Knives* listed at the end of Chapter 5. These are just a few ideas for jump-starting an eating plan. You can also use Dr. Google to find a gazillion others by their place on the diabetes teeter-totter.

You'll also need to plot macronutrients, particularly if a recipe doesn't include a macro composition, or if you wish to add food that's not part of a recipe. Fortunately, there are also a gazillion macro plotters available to help you do this. Some are free. My favorite is FatSecret (fatsecret.com). Other good programs are Lose It! (loseit.com), My Macros+ (getmymacros.com), and MyFitnessPal (myfitnesspal.com/food/search). These sites focus on weight loss and are hung up on the calorie-deficit model, but

---

† Nathan Pritikin was an American inventor, engineer, nutritionist, and longevity researcher who popularized the first high-carb, plant-based, very low-fat diet. He died in 1985, purportedly with a near-absence of cardiovascular disease.

no worries. Just enter your current weight as a goal weight or pick a lower weight that encapsulates the permanent five-hundred-calorie deficit mentioned previously.

A formal food plan won't be necessary for long, and once you get rolling, calories won't be as important. Healthy blood sugar numbers on a glucometer or CGM, using less insulin and fewer, if any, other diabetes medications, drive what you eat, not calories. You'll soon learn approximations, and consistent with the National Weight Control Registry research findings and the six rules of healthy diabetic eating, the process becomes easier, since your diet will be less varied and probably not as plentiful. As Dr. Bernstein says, "You will get into the habit of eating a certain way, into the habit of eating a certain amount, and over time it will all become second nature."[14]

Heuristics—cognitive shortcuts—help with approximations and play a role in getting to the place described by Dr. Bernstein. Food-related examples include eating oysters harvested only during months ending in "r" (to avoid food poisoning from eating warm-water oysters during spring and summer months), "An apple a day keeps the doctor away" (a reminder to eat whole fruit), and "Don't eat snacks after 6:00 p.m." (to allay blood sugar spikes while sleeping).

Author Michael Pollan's delightful *Food Rules: An Eater's Manual* includes many dietary heuristics, such as "The whiter the bread, the sooner you'll be dead" (#42) and "Make water your beverage of choice" (#40). A favorite of mine from Mr. Pollan is "Avoid food products with the word 'lite' or the terms 'low-fat' or 'nonfat' in their names" (#9).[15]

To conclude, with a plank on the teeter-totter chosen, the rules of healthy diabetic eating embedded and followed by the design and practice of a sustaining diet with manageable macronutrient proportions, you've launched into a much healthier future!

Exercise is next as we move up the hierarchy from what's most important to emphasize to what should be the least.

Dr. Jody Stanislaw Weighs In on Nutrition

What should I eat? This can be a constant dilemma for a person with diabetes. But as Chad describes in the previous chapters, the choice does not have to be so tough. Low carb is the way to go.

THE BENEFITS OF LOW-CARB EATING

Low carb done correctly is a very healthy diet. Plus, most importantly for people with diabetes, it makes keeping blood sugars in the optimal range much more easily achieved.

Chad's six rules of healthy diabetic eating and his macronutrient teeter-totter are based on sound nutritional concepts. (I do disagree slightly with one of the rules, which I reveal later.) Conversely, for those who are insulin-dependent, conventional medicine teaches that as long as the insulin-to-carb ratio is known, pretty much anything can be eaten. This does not work if your goal is to achieve healthy blood sugars! Dosing, to stay in range during *and after* the meal, is much more complex than any simple formula could accurately or regularly predict.

For example, dosing insulin for 15 grams of carb from eating an apple requires a different approach than dosing for 15 grams of carbs from eating black beans. Although an apple is a low-glycemic-index fruit, it can still quickly spike blood sugar, and thus a considerable amount of insulin must be dispensed before the apple is eaten. Beans, which not only contain complex carbs but are also full of protein, fat, and fiber, release glucose much more slowly. So diabetics consuming beans likely require half of their insulin dose up front and the other half perhaps an hour later.

This *timing* of dosing, something that is rarely taught, is a key skill that must be nuanced at every meal. *When low-carb meals are chosen, this complex problem of dosing becomes simpler, with less margin for error.*

Furthermore, when eating protein and fat with carbs (which is most often the case), the insulin-to-carb ratio can rarely even be valid. Protein itself can slowly raise blood sugar for approximately five hours. High fat can create temporary insulin resistance that can last for six hours, eight hours, or even longer. The more fat that is consumed, the longer that fat's effect on blood sugar lasts, *especially when combined with a lot of carbs.* Consequently, for those who are insulin-dependent, giving an extended bolus or multiple small doses over several hours is needed to cover high-fat meals. And fast-acting insulin isn't even fast enough to cover the speed of glucose absorption caused by high-carb choices.

Those who have T2D with functioning islet cells will experience these same issues with insulin resistance, glycemic variability, and potential adverse health effects as those with

continued

T1D, particularly if they combine high-fat *and* high-carb eating in what Chad refers to as the dietary "deadly duo."

At the root of the problem is the conventional eat-what-ever-you-want-and-cover-it-with-medication thinking; basically, treating food with medicine, whether it's insulin or pills. This thinking leads to poor health and is potentially life-threatening.

When I volunteer at diabetes summer camps where conventional eating is taught, I see this tragedy daily. The children count up their carbs from their pancakes and syrup, give themselves a huge dose of insulin, and then during the post-breakfast flag-football game, staff run around handing out glucose tabs. One year, I even witnessed a young girl have a seizure. The sad reality is that the majority of insulin-dependent children and many adults live this tragic eat-what-you-want-and-then-medicate lifestyle.

I have taught the benefits of eating low carb to hundreds of patients. Many have had diabetes for decades and yet have never been presented with the option to eat low carb. After just a few weeks of this new way of eating, my patients' glucose numbers dramatically improve.

Susan had A1cs in the 7s and 8s for thirty years. She suffered from retinopathy issues countless times. After her first three months of eating low carb, her A1c reached 5.9 percent, and she has had no retinopathy issues since. Rob is a police officer who thought he had to always stay with a blood sugar at 200 to avoid a low in case he had to suddenly run after a suspect. After Rob started eating low carb, his A1cs are now regularly in the low 5s.

The fact that the American Diabetes Association suggests an A1c goal of only below 7 percent, which equates to unhealthy average blood glucose of 154, is baffling to me. Perhaps it has to do with the fact that healthy A1cs cannot be reached on the Standard American Diet (SAD). Unfortunately, the SAD is full of "fake foods."

AVOID FAKE FOODS

Fake foods are usually very high carb, with an endless list of added sugars. They are items that are never found growing in nature. Fake foods have long ingredient lists, always containing many unknown substances that are extremely hard to even pronounce.

Real food comes from nature. Real food does not need a label. Real food is packed full of vitamins and nutrients that benefit your health. Chad's Rule 5 of healthy eating is all about eating real food. Eating real food reduces the risk of the greatest threat to the health of someone with diabetes: heart disease. Real food can also reduce the risk of some cancers, as well as reverse or at least reduce the severity or risk of type 2 diabetes. You can read twenty-one more benefits of eating real food here: healthline.com/nutrition/21-reasons-to-eat-real-food.

If you need help transforming your diet, the next time you go to the grocery store, start buying more vegetables and fewer fake foods. Reduce buying things that come in a box or a package. The next step could be to go on the internet to find whole food, low-carb recipes and then give them a try.

continued

DEALING WITH EMOTIONS

Having said all of this, any discussion of the proper diet must also address the emotional aspects of food. (I applaud Chad for flipping the current hierarchy of diabetes care and putting the mental part first.) If eating healthy was as easy as just eating real food and saying "no" to the fake foods, everyone would be doing it. Food is a touchy subject for many. There are strong family and cultural traditions as well as emotional reasons for eating.

Personally, after having to weigh and measure every bite of food I ate starting when I was diagnosed at the age of seven, I developed an eating disorder in my teens. I was so full of rebellion that I couldn't handle following any more rules about what I could and could not eat.

How did I eventually find peace? By allowing myself the thought that I *could* eat anything I want, anytime I want. If I want a freshly baked cookie (my favorite treat of all time), I will let myself have it. The good news is that with this open-minded approach of no "off-limits" foods, I actually rarely want the fake foods now. This approach works for hundreds of my patients as well.

This works because no human likes to be told what to do. When we are, resentment and rebellion often surface. Furthermore, when we're given the freedom to choose, most gravitate to what makes us feel the best in the long run. This is why I must disagree with Chad's rule 4 of the six rules of healthy diabetic eating—that certain foods should be forbidden.

My disagreement with Chad comes with an important

qualification. Eating fake or junk food can never be an everyday habit. If you limit your forbidden foods to, let's say, once a month, there's little risk to overall health, but only if those who are insulin-dependent are also well-skilled in how to dose fake or junk food safely and effectively.

My last point is one that is sadly often forgotten— eating food can and should be *pleasurable*. It is important that you find the balance between not only what's best for your body but what you enjoy and what makes you feel good. Don't try to follow a diet just because you think you should. Avoid extremes and absolutes.

If this real-food, low-carb approach is totally new to you, have patience. Take baby steps toward what is healthier and away from high-carb, fake foods. Over time, your taste buds will change. Have patience and determination. Eventually, you'll discover the intersection between what is healthy and what is joyful. By adopting a diet of real food that is low carb, my hope for you is that you will achieve the best blood sugars of your life.

*   *   *

Dr. Jody Stanislaw received her doctorate in naturopathic medicine in 2007, is a certified diabetes care and education specialist, and has lived with type 1 diabetes herself since the age of seven. From her more than thirty-five years of experience, she teaches life-changing information about how to successfully manage T1D that standard medical care rarely teaches. She runs a virtual consulting practice

continued

and thus works with individuals with T1D located around the world. In addition to focusing on improving one's diabetes, she also supports patients with diet, exercise, sleep, and emotional health.

Dr. Stanislaw has a series of virtual training courses that cover how to avoid the blood sugar roller-coaster, dose properly, why carb counting doesn't work, mastering blood sugar during exercise, and how to stay positive and avoid burnout. Her latest project is a virtual membership program called the T1D Crew, a supportive and educational space for those with T1D. Her TEDx talk, "Sugar Is Not a Treat," has over two million views (go to drjodynd.com to learn more). Those with T1D who are interested in a free consultation with Dr. Stanislaw can visit drjodynd.com/consultation.

Questions for Your Care Providers

- *How many calories should I eat each day and how did you determine this number?*

- *What eating rules or guidelines do you recommend?*
  (You could discuss here the six rules of healthy diabetic eating outlined in Chapter 5.)

- *How much protein should I consume daily?*

And questions for the reader:

- *What are three dietary heuristics that will help you eat more healthily?*

- *How much daily fiber did you typically consume over, say, three days? (You could use an app recommended in the chapter to determine this.) How might you increase this amount?*

Further Reading

BOOKS

- Bailor, Jonathan. *The Calorie Myth: How to Eat More, Exercise Less, Lose Weight, and Live Better.* New York: Harper Wave, 2014.

- Burkitt, Denis Parsons. *Don't Forget Fibre in Your Diet: To Help Avoid Many of Our Commonest Diseases.* London: Collins, 1979. (This forty-year-old classic by the "Fiber Man" is still good reading today. It's out of print but still available on Amazon and AbeBooks.)

- Collen, Alanna. *10% Human: How Your Body's Microbes Hold the Key to Health and Happiness.* New York: HarperCollins, 2015. (A well-written and researched exploration of the microbiome, gut bacteria, and fungi that benefit from fiber.)

- Pollan, Michael. *Food Rules: An Eater's Manual.* New York: Penguin Books, 2011.

OTHER RESOURCES

For a concise list of the best weight-loss and nutrition apps according to *Prevention*, visit prevention.com/weight-loss/a20468312/best-weight-loss-apps.

CHAPTER 7

MAKING SENSE OF EXERCISE

The benefits of exercise are overwhelming. Here's a representative list from the American Heart Association (AHA), all convincingly supported by research:

- Lower risk of heart disease, stroke, type 2 diabetes, high blood pressure, dementia and Alzheimer's, several types of cancer, and some complications of pregnancy.

- Better sleep, including improvements in insomnia and obstructive sleep apnea.

- Improved cognition, including memory, attention, and processing speed.

- Less weight gain, obesity, and related chronic health conditions.

- Better balance and bone health, with less risk of injury from falls.

- Fewer symptoms of depression and anxiety.

- Better quality of life and sense of overall well-being.[1]

For those with diabetes, exercise also significantly reduces A1c values, lowers insulin resistance whether the insulin is injected, endogenous, or a combination thereof, and improves other markers of metabolic syndrome.[2] It also plays a crucial role in helping safely maintain healthy blood sugars using a minimum of medication.

How much exercise and what types are enough? The answers, found in places such as the AHA and the ADA websites, are derived from the US Department of Health and Human Services recommendations published in a 2018 second-edition report.[3] Adults need a minimum of 150 minutes of moderately intense exercise *or* 75 minutes of vigorous-intensity aerobic exercise each week. Preferably, this activity is spread throughout the week. In addition, muscle-strengthening activities of moderate or greater intensity should occur on two or more nonconcurrent days a week.

Government-recommended minimums for those with chronic conditions are the same as for able-bodied people. If an adult with a chronic condition, such as diabetes, is unable to meet the minimums, the guidelines call for them to still engage in regular physical activity according to their abilities and to avoid inactivity.

Exercise Considerations

Misconceptions about exercise abound, any of which is a barrier to creating and sustaining a successful exercise program.

DON'T TRY TO LOSE WEIGHT BY EXERCISING

Trying to lose weight through exercise is futile. The math of caloric deficit is part of the problem. A 170-pound man who runs thirty minutes on an elliptical machine burns only 347 calories, about the number in a jelly donut. He'd have to walk for about ninety minutes to use up the same number of calories.[4] Is he going to spend all this time and effort to eat one jelly donut? The answer, of course, is no. But he'll still eat the donut!

A related conundrum is that nutrition and exercise are two sides of the same good-health coin. We need *both* to establish and maintain healthy metabolic homeostasis. One won't effectively offset the other. It's not surprising, then, that exercise by itself usually doesn't contribute meaningfully to healthy, sustained weight loss.[5] For example, exercise sustained at a moderate to intensive level *for over an hour each day* only leads to the possibility of small weight loss.[6] That much exercise for that little of a result is not realistic or likely for most people.

The big weight losses from unhealthy temporary exceptions—say, from the agony of contestants on a reality television show or quick weight loss from intense exercise for hours in the gym coupled with yo-yo dieting—don't count and shouldn't be taken seriously.

However, sustaining a regular exercise program for health, to the extent that it contributes to healthy physiological homeostasis, is necessary and useful for *maintaining* weight loss around a healthy set point.

YOU DON'T HAVE TO JOIN A GYM

Despite what the $30 billion health and fitness industry in the United States would have you believe, you don't have to join a fitness club or gym. There are benefits to a gym membership if you prefer to use a wide range of exercise machines or want on-site help using them or otherwise designing a program. But you can easily exercise at home using a treadmill or an elliptical machine picked up cheaply at a garage sale, as well as your body weight and a set of dumbbells for resistance training.

YOU DON'T HAVE TO SWEAT BUCKETS FOR HOURS

Thankfully, exercising for health doesn't take a lot of time. The weekly 75 minutes to 150 minutes, with some resistance training folded in, isn't much, and it can be conveniently distributed throughout the 168 hours of the week, although more intense exercise sessions shouldn't be scheduled on concurrent days.

It's surprising how much benefit comes from even just a little bit of exercise. In one study, just a few minutes of focused exercise each day decreased mortality up to 22 percent in older adults.[7] In another study, walking just four thousand to eight thousand steps per day (far short of the proverbial ten thousand) still cut the risk of cancer or heart disease death by two-thirds.[8]

YOU DON'T HAVE TO LIKE IT

Some experts think we'll quit exercising if we're not having fun. Here's an example offered by diabetes exercise expert Dr. Sheri Colberg:

One thing people forget to consider when designing a fitness program is enjoyment. Do you think the people you see grunting and groaning during agonizing workouts are truly enjoying themselves? Due to human nature, if the activities you pick are simply not fun for you, you're likely to stop doing them at some point.[9]

There's even been a call to rebrand exercise for those with diabetes as fun rather than as a chore.[10] Then, supposedly, we might do more of it.

That's just not a realistic view. Expectancy theory, covered in Chapter 3, helps explain why. You might recall that the theory deals with multiplicative factors that drive the force of motivation, all three of which have to be high for motivation to be high. If you haven't enjoyed exercise in the past, your first-level expectancy—the belief that your effort will lead to performance (that exercising will be fun)—will be extremely low (let's say only 10 percent on a scale of 0 to 100 percent). However, you're 100 percent sure that exercise will make you healthy (instrumentality, a second-level expectancy) and 100 percent sure that you value good health (valence). Despite strong instrumentality and valence, your force of motivation is still low: $10\% \times 100\% \times 100\% =$ only 10%, just one-tenth of total motivation possible. You're doomed from the start.

But the math changes if you begin with a different expectation. Start out viewing exercise for health as a chore, and don't expect to have fun. Think of it as a chore you accomplish regularly, like mowing the lawn. Sometimes you don't get to it on time, but it still gets done. Let's say in percentage terms that you're 80 percent sure that you'll get the lawn cut every week, about a two-and-a-half-hour job. Ditto spending that same time every week doing exercise. Extrapolating from the previous numbers in this example, your force of motivation to exercise for health jumps from 10 percent to 80 percent: 80% × 100% × 100% = 80%.

This math works for me. I'd be defeated right from the start if I expected exercising for health to be fun. I don't like running on an elliptical machine or lifting weights. But then, I don't expect to have fun when I do these things, making the issue moot. Instead, I view exercising for health the same way I do other rote activities of daily life that I'm pretty sure I can complete, such as mowing the lawn, brushing my teeth, taking showers, or injecting insulin and changing CGM sensors. It's something on the schedule that's not fun but necessary. Thankfully—and this is key—you don't have to do a lot of it.

This doesn't mean that all exercise has to be drudgery. But the two purposes of exercise—for health and fun—should be kept separate. For example, I love playing golf. I'll play eighteen holes, but then I still have to complete my regular twenty-five-minute aerobic workout when I get home because it's Wednesday.*

Another way to think about the distinction is to view exercise for fun as a leisure-time activity. It could be spent playing golf which, coincidentally, is exercise, but this time could also be spent as a couch potato playing video games or reading a book. It's that little bit of focused and goal-directed exercise for health that truly matters, and that must happen on a regular, scheduled basis.

What if you're the rare person who genuinely has fun running on an elliptical machine and lifting weights? Bonus! You

---

* For me, golf isn't exercising for health because it lacks the focus and intensity to meet the US Department of Health and Human Services' and my fitness goals. Plus, it can take four-and-a-half hours to play a round. I'm not doing anything for that long unless it's fun!

kill the exercise for health and fun birds with one stone. The rest of us aren't so lucky. (I suppose I could transform golfing for fun into exercise for health by playing cardio golf, running from ball to ball down each fairway, but I prefer walking or riding in a cart.)

Realizing that you don't have to like exercising for health but still need to do it also fits into the mold of realizing that a diabetic metabolism isn't normal—that good health begins with maintaining a twelve-step perspective, adhering to a nutritional plank on the diabetes teeter-totter, and following the six rules of healthy diabetic eating. It's just the way it is.

Making Exercise Happen

On to creating a program! Safety comes first. The next steps are designing, scheduling, and implementing your workouts.

SAFETY IS PARAMOUNT

Realistically assessing physical capacities comes first. Initially, even light exercise may be overwhelming or too stressful for your joints. Diabetes complications can also be an issue. Retinopathy, neuropathy, kidney disease, or cardiovascular disease may pose limitations that mandate a conversation with your care provider.

The second major safety issue concerns the blood-sugar-lowering effect of exercise. Intense cardio can burn upward of 100 grams of glucose per hour![11] Consequently, combining exercise and blood-sugar-lowering medications can be unsafe, even life-threatening (see Table 7.1 for a list of these medications). Eating fast-acting carbs before exercising, lowering your basal rate on an insulin pump, or doing both is usually a good, safe idea—but with an important exception.

Table 7.1. Blood-sugar-lowering medications

Any type of insulin

Rapid-acting: glulisine (Apidra), lispro (Humalog, Admelog), lispro aabc (Lyumjev), aspart (Novolog), aspart recombinant (Fiasp)

Short-acting: regular (Humulin R, Novolin R), Humulin U-500

Intermediate-acting: NPH (Humulin N, Novolin N)

Long-acting: detemir (Levemir), glargine U-100 (Lantus, Basaglar, Semglee)

Ultra-long-acting: glargine U-300 (Toujeo), degludec (Tresiba)

Combinations/premixed insulins

Inhaled insulin: insulin human powder (Afrezza)

Sulfonylureas

Glimepiride (Amaryl)

Glyburide (DiaBeta)

Chlorpropamide (Diabinese)

Glipizide (Glucotrol)

Glyburide micronized (Glynase)

continued

Glyburide (Micronase)

Tolbutamide (Orinase)

Tolazamide (Tolinase)

Meglitinides

Nateglinide (Starlix)

Repaglinide (Prandin)

Thanks go to Ginger Vieira for providing this list.

Sometimes the opposite occurs. Those who are insulin-dependent might experience *hyperglycemia* if they eat fast-acting carbs before a heavy, intense anaerobic workout. They might even experience hyperglycemia without the carbs. Stress from strenuous exercise and associated muscle strain releases hormones such as glucagon and epinephrine into the bloodstream. These hormones, in turn, signal the liver and muscles to dump stored glucose, an amount that can overwhelm available insulin and send blood sugar skyrocketing.

Exercising with high blood sugar above 250 mg/dL by itself is also dangerous. Your blood sugar is already too high, and if it escalates from there as described above, you could start on the road to diabetic ketoacidosis. You should use test strips to check for ketone bodies in your urine or blood. If they're present, avoid exercise until ketones are absent and your blood sugar has fallen.[12]

If you use blood-sugar-lowering medications, it's important to work with your care provider to figure out the glycemic effects of your exercise program. From there, and again with the help of your care provider, refine your treatment strategies accordingly. For example, I have to eat 16 grams of dextrose tabs before a twenty-five-minute cardio session because my blood sugar drops like a rock. Conversely, the diabetes writer and former competitive powerlifter Ginger Vieira occasionally requires a small bolus after a heavy-resistance workout because stress-induced hormones cause her blood sugars to *rise*.[13]

Of course, all adjustments depend on your starting blood sugar level. These are merely representative examples, and there are many more. For example, if you're doing a strenuous activity like racquetball with a starting blood sugar under 100 mg/dL, you might be advised to eat 50 carb grams per hour and to monitor your glucose carefully.[14]

Safety-related questions to your care providers, then, are: How much and what type of exercise can I safely handle? What will my proposed exercise program do to my blood sugar? And how do I deal with it?

DESIGNING A WORKOUT

I begin this subject by further defining the types of exercise mentioned throughout this chapter.

Aerobic exercise, also referred to as "cardio," causes breathing and pulse rates to increase for a sustained time. Swimming laps, jogging, fast walking on a treadmill, and cycling are examples. *Anaerobic exercise* involves quick bursts of energy during which muscles are stressed and maximum effort is expended for a short time. Examples include resistance training such as lifting with heavy weights and sprinting. High-intensity interval training, or HIIT, involving short, repeated cycles of strenuous exercise followed by brief rest periods is another example of anaerobic exercise.

It's possible to move between exercise types. In this regard, aerobic exercise can be made anaerobic by ramping up the intensity. A way to know that this line has been crossed is when you *suddenly* can't breathe after sprinting the last 100 yards of a long, slow aerobic run and end up with your hands on your knees, panting anaerobically.

Both types of exercise are important. Aerobic cardio significantly improves cardiovascular function and all markers for metabolic health. Anaerobic resistance training builds stronger bones and muscles and improves balance. Consequently, a weekly exercise schedule should incorporate both. However, this may not be possible right away if your conditioning doesn't allow it. You may need to start aerobically by only walking around the block four times a week and doing light weights on a couple of other days. Then, build up to include anaerobic resistance exercise later.

Regular, structured exercise is dynamic. Regardless of your starting place, you can expect to see improvements in conditioning and strength over time. Adjusting your workouts in response to improvement is a healthy option. You might still do the two-and-a-half hours of moderately intense exercise or seventy-five minutes of vigorous exercise weekly, but perhaps at a faster pace. The two nonconcurrent, weekly resistance sessions might be done with more weight. If you're the rare individual who likes exercise as an end in itself, you might even expand to five hours a week, the maximum recommended in government guidelines.

A plethora of resources exists for designing your first workout program and for tweaking it as time goes by with the help of your care provider. Just as a ton of recipe books exist for cooking, there are equally as many exercise books, typically showing an incredibly fit person going through the paces of a preferred routine. The diabetes periodicals listed at the end of Chapter 1, such as *Diabetes Self-Management*, frequently display routines with their articles on exercise.

You can also hire a personal trainer. If you've joined a gym, there might be one available at little or no extra cost. Your care provider might also recommend an exercise physiologist, which is a step up from a personal trainer. If you seek an expert's help, make sure they thoroughly understand diabetes in general and your specific needs in particular. You might also consider checking first to see if they're certified by an organization such as the American Council on Exercise (ACE) or the National Academy of Sports Medicine (NASM). Shop around. And again, make sure your care provider is always okay with your exercise program at whatever its stage of evolution.

You can consult one of the many apps available that address nutrition and exercise. I listed a few in Chapter 6 such as MyFitnessPal and Lose It! These apps are excellent. However, it might be better to choose one that pertains just to exercise. Sworkit might fit the bill for you (sworkit.com). My favorite, however, is the Johnson & Johnson Official 7 Minute Workout, one of the earliest exercise apps developed (7minuteworkout.jnj.com).

No gym or exercise equipment is necessary with the Johnson & Johnson app. Beginner through advanced aerobic and anaerobic routines are combined so you can exercise at home with your body weight as resistance. Only twenty-one minutes are needed to complete three circuits during each workout. Do this four days a week, and you're past the seventy-five-minute, vigorous-intensity threshold called for in government guidelines.

SCHEDULING EXERCISE FOR HEALTH

You could do the Johnson & Johnson routine for the combined forty-two minutes, two days a week, and still hit the mark. It's not necessary to schedule workouts with identical time intervals as long as you get the time in, and as long as the intense-resistance exercise isn't scheduled on consecutive days so you can let your muscles rest.

Regardless of how it's configured, it's important to schedule exercise consistently and then stick to that schedule, treating exercise for health as a necessary chore. For example, I brush and floss my teeth every evening at about the same time. I exercise at the same time every day as well, for twenty-five minutes, six days a week, at about 4:00 p.m., alternating cardio and resistance. I take Sunday off because it's the end of my week.

How to coordinate exercise and meals? A person with type 2 diabetes who doesn't use insulin or other blood sugar-lowering medication might schedule exercise an hour *after* a meal. Doing so, at least for the meal in question, improves insulin sensitivity and blunts the inevitable after-meal blood sugar spike in those with insulin resistance.[15]

However, if you use blood sugar-lowering medication, it might be best to exercise *before* a meal. Consider doing fasted exercise before breakfast or in the afternoon before dinner, letting at least four hours go by between a meal and working out. This simplifies things with no bolus insulin or carbs from a recent meal in play. However, beware of fasted exercise while doing strenuous anaerobic exercise with little insulin on board. As mentioned, this may lead to a significant blood sugar spike. Either develop a plan for covering a rapid rise in this situation or stick to aerobic cardio when doing fasted exercise.

Time to move on! The next chapter on drugs and devices completes the hierarchy of diabetes care as it should be.

Delaine Wright Weighs In on Exercise

I'm one of the lucky people mentioned by Chad who generally likes to exercise (especially when I have my favorite tunes to help me keep the beat!). But in my twenty-seven-year career as a clinical exercise physiologist and certified diabetes educator who is living actively with type 1 herself, I have also worked closely with people who felt the exact opposite—so I understand and empathize completely. And I will also admit that I've experienced times in my life when I fell away from my exercise routine, lost the "like," and had to fight a bit to return to and embrace it again. So I *do* appreciate Chad's approach of seeing exercise as a chore that we each just *have* to do—like brushing our teeth or mowing the lawn.

I also want to emphasize that it is important to "prep the way" by reducing as many individual barriers as possible. Part of that behavioral process involves knowing yourself and then making it as *easy* as possible for you to choose exercise over skipping a workout. For example, some of us do best when we exercise at a particular time of day, when it's easiest to avoid other things getting in the way—"getting it behind us" first thing in the morning, for example.

continued

Exercising with a friend or partner is another "trick" that can help—misery loves company, as they say—and you'll feel a little guilty perhaps if you don't show up at your neighbor's front door for that daily walk. Signing up for a paid class or a paid scheduled workout with a personal trainer is another method to keep you on track. Schedule it into your calendar and set that reminder alarm on your phone. Perhaps your music playlist is what motivates *you* to move your feet to a beat—nothing wrong with that at all. Place your sneakers and workout wear by the door so it's the first thing you see when you return to your house at the end of the day. Spend some thinking time figuring out what you need to do to "make it easy to happen" with exercise and then put it into practice.

Staying on top of blood sugar when you exercise is important. I always encourage people with diabetes to run a blood sugar experiment by testing (or tracking CGM data) before, during, and after exercise. Take good notes on what your exercise routine was like for the session. Be your own science project! It can be eye-opening. Not only will keeping track help you balance your blood sugar levels around exercise, but it's also *so* empowering to see the difference that even thirty minutes of exercise can make on your levels! It's so powerful a benefit that you're often that much more motivated to do it again the next day.

And if you're someone who struggles a bit with the hypoglycemia (low blood sugar) associated with exercise, you'll learn what your body needs to avoid a low. As an active person with type 1 diabetes, I know how frustrating it can be to have to shove food in your mouth so that you can exercise. Once I understood my own glycemic response to exercise, I worked with my health care team, endocrinologist, and diabetes educator to adjust my basal insulin flow to avoid *having* to eat to exercise. And as a diabetes health care professional, I've helped many others do the same.

Throughout my career, I've had the opportunity to work with many high-level endurance athletes who excelled at their sport despite, and I would also say *because of*, diabetes. A triathlete with type 1 diabetes who has the eventual goal of completing the Ironman Triathlon (which consists of a 2.4-mile swim, a 112-mile bike ride, and a marathon 26.22-mile run, raced consecutively in that order) must learn their individual blood sugar response to various training workouts. The adjustments that need to be made to manage blood sugars around exercise differ significantly when completing a training run versus a swim. And as the workloads, duration, and distance increase over weeks and months, so too do the required adjustments to both insulin levels and fuel intake. An athlete with diabetes develops this incredible understanding and puts it into practice during every workout.

As Chad has pointed out, even for those not training for endurance events, different types of exercise activities and varying intensities can drastically affect the glycemic response. That's where patterning and being a good observer, notetaker, and researcher will help you understand what is going on in your particular situation—and allow you to make adaptations that work for you.

continued

Also, remember that it's not just formal exercise that demonstrates an impressive blood glucose response. Even simple activities around the house that involve movement (such as doing housework or working in the yard) can also significantly lower blood sugar. And this positive benefit can last for hours. Do this tracking experiment by testing and patterning your blood sugars around everyday activities—this *will* help motivate you to move more! We have a lot of positive power in our own two hands and our own two feet. Every little bit helps, in more ways than one.

And last, I would say that even though you might not be someone who finds exercise fun right now, I promise that you *can* find some fun in exercise! Occasionally, make it an adventure to do something different. Plan a walk (or a more strenuous hike) somewhere that you haven't necessarily been before. Embrace nature and the outdoors. Learn a new skill, try something different, challenge yourself, create some memories, have some laughs, or enjoy your family, grandkids, and friends in an adventuresome new way.

Allow a life with diabetes to activate and empower you to live your life *fully*—and you'll have a positive, motivating, and inspirational effect on so many others around you as well!

* * *

Delaine Wright is a master's-level clinical exercise physiologist who has spent a rewarding twenty-seven-year career in health care working as a certified diabetes educator and team lead of a hospital-based cardiac and pulmonary rehabilitation and wellness program in southern Rhode Island. She lives actively with type 1 diabetes herself, having been diagnosed at age fifteen in 1983.

Delaine was an early member of the famous Children with Diabetes (CWD) DTeam, answering questions in an online support system. She has appeared on episodes of the *DLife* television series, sharing her story of participation in aerial arts while managing blood sugars in the air. She was a founding member of the Fit4D (now Cecelia Health) team of diabetes professionals that provides personal coaching for those living with diabetes. In this role, she has coached a wide variety of athletes with diabetes—including marathoners, cyclists, swimmers, triathletes, and even other aerialists.

Delaine has lectured nationally to PWDs and health care professionals on diabetes management and exercise, as well as cardiovascular disease prevention and wellness. She has written articles and shared her expertise in books and publications over the years. She is honored to add a voice to Chad's publication.

Questions for Your Care Providers

- *What exercise regimen do you recommend considering my medical history and why?* This will be an ongoing question as your exercise routine evolves.

- *What will my proposed exercise program do to my blood sugar? Will it spike it? Lower it?* Much depends here on the type of exercise you plan, the time of day, and timing with meals. You shouldn't just assume exercise will lower blood sugar.

- *How do I deal with changes in blood sugar during and immediately after exercise?* Your care provider might provide you with a detailed chart that correlates different exercise types and intensities with blood sugars and needed carb or medication levels, or they might keep the communication simpler. Either way, make sure you're comfortable with their recommendations.

Further Reading

BOOKS

- Bernstein, Richard K. "Using Exercise to Enhance Insulin Sensitivity." In *Dr. Bernstein's Diabetes Solution: The Complete Guide to Achieving Normal Blood Sugars*, chap. 14. New York: Little, Brown Spark, 2011.

- Colberg, Sheri R. *Diabetic Athlete's Handbook*. Champaign, IL: Human Kinetics, 2009.

- Colberg, Sheri R., and the American Diabetes Association. *Diabetes and Keeping Fit for Dummies*. Hoboken, NJ: Wiley, 2018. (Dr. Colberg is one of the leading authorities on diabetes and exercise in the United States.)

- Oerum, Christel. *Fit with Diabetes*. Self-published, 2018. (This ebook can be downloaded at diabetesstrong.com/ fit-with-diabetes. Oerum's book has specific information for those with T1D but is still worthwhile reading for those with T2D.)

OTHER RESOURCES

- Bolus and Barbells: bolusandbarbells.org. This website is a good information source for those with T1D interested in strength training.

- *Diabetes Strong*: diabetesstrong.com. This site has nutrition, exercise, and general info for all of us.

- Ginger Vieira: gingervieira.com and youtube.com/user/ gingervieira/featured. (A special plug here for Ginger Vieira, who's had T1D for over twenty years. Ginger has certifications in cognitive coaching and personal training, among others. Although we don't always agree, if I had a diabetes coach, it'd be Ginger!)

- The Johnson & Johnson Official 7-Minute Workout: 7minuteworkout.jnj.com. A great program!

CHAPTER 8

MAKING SENSE OF DRUGS AND DEVICES

Don't get me wrong—we need some drugs and devices. Insulin is a lifesaver for people with type 1 diabetes. Blood sugar-monitoring technologies are crucial for all. But there otherwise has been too much emphasis on oral medications, insulins, other injectables, and technologies relative to the benefits of getting the mental part right (such as practicing a twelve-step perspective), practicing good nutrition, and exercising, which are truly foundational to our good health. That's why drugs and devices are covered last in this book; they are the least important in the hierarchy of diabetes care as it should be.

Too Much

Prescription medications pervade American society, overwhelmingly so in the treatment of diabetes, particularly T2D. The development of new medications and devices rolls on unabated. As noted in Chapter 2, the 2020 *Diabetes Forecast* special edition on medications and devices touted more than 240 available, a 60 percent increase in just two years!

When diabetes entered my life in 1968, there was just one class of diabetes medication other than insulin: the sulfonylureas. Today, there are eleven different classes, not counting myriad forms of insulin: sulfonylureas, meglitinides, biguanides (metformin), thiazolidinediones (TZDs), glucosidase inhibitors, glucagon-like peptide-1 receptor agonists (GLP-1s), dipeptidyl peptidase 4 (DPP-4) inhibitors, amylin analogs, a dopamine agonist (bromocriptine), a bile acid sequestrant (colesevelam), and sodium-glucose cotransporter-2 (SGLT-2) inhibitors.[1] Most of these classes have many generic and branded products included in them. Then, there are the seven types of insulin listed in Chapter 7 (Table 7.1).

There are also at least eighteen medications that *combine* drugs from these varied classes. For example, alogliptin, a DPP-4 inhibitor, is combined with metformin in a branded product, Kazano. Empagliflozin, an SGLT-2 inhibitor, combines with linagliptin, a DPP-4 inhibitor, to become Glyxambi, and pioglitazone, a TZD, joins glimepiride, a sulfonylurea, to become Duetact. Qternmet combines three diabetes medications: dapagliflozin, an SGLT-2 inhibitor; saxagliptin, a DPP-4 inhibitor; and metformin.

Many people with T2D take several of these medications simultaneously, including combination medications. Some also include bolus or basal insulin or both in the mix. Consequently, it's not surprising that the most common contributor to polypharmacy in the United States, defined as taking five or more medications daily, is T2D medications.[2] It's also not surprising that "the potential permutations of various combinations of these agents is staggering and can be bewildering to the clinicians trying to design the optimum therapy regimen for a given patient."[3]

Those with T1D aren't immune to polypharmacy. Besides insulin, some are also prescribed a GLP-1 agonist or an SGLT-2 inhibitor. About 1 percent of those with T1D also inject an amylin analog. Amylin is a pancreatic hormone that is absent in those with T1D and impaired in many with T2D. It complements the after-meal action of insulin in a healthy metabolism by turning down another hormone, glucagon, that tells the liver to release sugar. A barrier to its use as a medication is the hassle of extra injections because it's incompatible in the same syringe with insulin. Stanford researchers recently discovered an elegant fix.[4] Yet another miracle on the way?

So whose fault is it that diabetes medications proliferate? The companies? Our care providers? Us? The companies are an easy target. After all, AstraZeneca, Merck, Eli Lilly, Novo Nordisk, and Sanofi exist to increase shareholder value. They do this by cranking out diabetes medications for sale to an increasingly diabetic marketplace. They also lobby. And they spend huge sums on advertising, leading to today's irrational juxtaposition of prime-time TV commercials for diabetes medications side by side with those for fast food and weight-loss programs.

However, it's unrealistic to expect Big Pharma and its supporting network to be, or to do, anything else. This leaves us with the responsibility for helping ourselves more and Big Pharma less by living in a way that minimizes our need for medication.

Less Is More

There are several benefits to focusing on nutrition and exercise rather than medication to safely maintain healthy blood sugars. Doing so eliminates or significantly reduces medication side effects and interactions. You'll also save a lot of money.

LESSEN SIDE EFFECTS

Every medication within the eleven classes and the seven insulins included in Table 7.1 come with potential side effects. The most dangerous is hypoglycemia for insulin, sulfonylurea, and meglitinide users. Weight gain is another side effect of these medications, but it pales in comparison to the threat of hypoglycemia.

Insulin and other blood sugar-lowering medications can be dangerous. Hypoglycemia causes 235,000 emergency-room trips each year in the United States.[5] In one study, one-third of adult subjects who experienced severe hypoglycemia died within three years from a heart attack or stroke.[6] (The reason for this wasn't clear, although cardiovascular stress from the event in question, and on other hypoglycemic occasions, probably contributed.) And 4 to 10 percent of all those with T1D die from hypoglycemia.[7]

Safely managing blood sugars with the smallest amounts of medication significantly reduces these threats. Otherwise, with big boluses come big variations in blood sugar, including downward, screaming drops on the glycemic roller coaster. To reiterate, Dr. Bernstein hit this nail on the head in observing that with big doses of insulin come big variation; small doses, small variation.[8]

The unpredictability of insulin is a problem in general, exacerbated by large doses. We're taught to bolus based on a static carb-to-insulin ratio. The reality is different not just because protein and fat also affect blood sugar but because insulin absorption differs. One study found a 10 to 20 percent variability in the absorption of short-acting insulin from one injection to the next.[9] Another study shows absorption variance up to 39 percent, depending on the injection site.[10]

And then, as discussed in Chapter 3, there are the forty-one other factors aside from insulin affecting blood sugar, such as fat and protein ingested with a meal, stress levels, exercise before eating, illness, how much sleep was gotten the night before, and the dawn effect in the morning when hormones elevate blood sugar.

Medications other than insulin are rife with side effects—so many that it's tempting to cherry-pick to make the point that less is more. Instead, I focus primarily on a recently introduced drug that I picked out of a hat: the SGLT-2 inhibitor dapagliflozin (brand name Farxiga). Approved by the FDA in 2013, dapagliflozin lowers blood sugar by passing excess glucose through the kidneys and urine.

In 2020, it was reported that dapagliflozin reduced kidney failure, heart failure hospitalization, and cardiovascular death in chronic kidney disease patients.[11] That's encouraging and shows that not all side effects are negative. However, the FDA had warned four years previously about the risk of acute kidney injury when taking the drug.[12] In 2015, this agency also warned of the risk associated with the use of SGLT-2 inhibitors of developing euglycemic diabetic ketoacidosis. Other potential side effects from the drug include increased urination or urgency, lower blood pressure, dizziness, genital yeast infections, urinary tract infections, increased blood potassium, and rare severe allergic reactions.[13]

That's just for one drug. Potential side effects come with all other medications. In this era of polypharmacy, it then becomes important to look at everything in the pillbox. For example, for someone with T2D, a physician might prescribe Xigduo XR, a brand name for a medication that combines dapagliflozin with the most prescribed of oral diabetes medications, metformin. Or the medications might be prescribed separately. In either case, the potential side effects list now grows to include those from metformin: diarrhea, gas, nausea, vitamin B12 depletion that could cause anemia, constipation, physical weakness, chest discomfort, and heartburn.[14]

These are the potential side effects of combining just two medications. Many with diabetes also take meds to treat other conditions, typically related to heart, blood pressure, or cholesterol issues, all with side effects of their own to add to the list.

LESSEN INTERACTIONS

To side effects can be added interactions. Coadministered drugs may interact in a way that alters the effectiveness or toxicity of any or all of them. In other words, they don't play well together. A particular food or an existing medical condition can also interact with a drug. Table 8.1 defines major, moderate, and minor interactions.

Table 8.1. Drug interactions

Major	Highly clinically significant. Avoid combinations; the risk of an interaction outweighs the benefit.
Moderate	Moderately clinically significant. Usually, avoid combinations; use only under special circumstances.
Minor	Minimally clinically significant. Minimize risk; assess risk and consider an alternative drug, take steps to circumvent the interaction risk, and/or institute a monitoring plan.

Source: Drugs.com "Drug Interactions Checker," drugs.com/drug_interactions.html.

A few examples: Dapagliflozin has a moderate interaction with alcohol, and major interactions are associated with renal deficiency and bladder cancer. The drug may also moderately interact with blood pressure in older patients. If metformin is added to the mix, there are additional major interactions with alcohol use and liver or kidney impairment to consider. Some of the interactions are surprising. For example, both drugs interact moderately with lisinopril, a frequently prescribed blood-pressure medication for those taking these diabetes medications.[15]

Keep in mind that side effects and interactions may not occur, might be tolerable if they do, or might be insignificant. A care provider prescribes a medication because in their professional judgment more benefit will occur than harm. That's as it should be. Our job is to make sure we understand the costs and benefits. You can also consult with your pharmacist if you have questions and bring concerns back to your care provider. Then it's up to you to decide what to do with the information.

Something to consider: The benefit of an SGLT-2 inhibitor, such as dapagliflozin, on blood sugar was only a 0.5 to 0.6 percent improvement in A1c in one study.[16] In another, even when dapagliflozin was added to two other oral diabetes medications, there was only a 1.0 percent improvement in A1c in subjects whose diabetes was "out of control."[17] Even after three medications, going from an average blood sugar of 212 mg/dL to 183 mg/dL is still significantly above the unhealthy cutoff of 140 mg/dL, and it did nothing to improve insulin resistance or stem unhealthy hyperinsulinemia in these subjects.

Is this slight benefit worth the cost in potential medication side effects and interactions? Probably not. But that's a call for you to make—again, in consultation with your care provider.

There are times when medical interventions work wonders that outweigh side effects and interactions. And I'm not just referring here to insulin for those with T1D. For example, bariatric surgery for people who are morbidly or significantly obese can put T2D in remission—80 percent in one study.[18] An emerging class of new injectable diabetes medication called dual GIP and GLP-1 receptor agonists, with tirzepatide as the first drug in the class, leads to significant weight loss and normalization of blood sugar in most people with T2D. The same is true of Wegovy, a reformulation of semaglutide, an injected GLP-1 receptor agonist. Combining drugs such as these with bariatric surgery can also have dramatic and positive multiplier effects on weight loss and blood sugars.

All well and good. However, in the absence of a healthy mindset, nutrition, and exercise, the problem remains how to *sustain* the weight loss and good health engendered by these interventions. There's also the cost, which may not be covered by insurance, especially for surgical interventions and new drugs such as tirzepatide and Wegovy.

SAVE MONEY

A healthy diet and exercise mean less medication and all the financial savings that go along with this. For some, it's a significant amount. In the United States, people with diabetes have $9,600 in annual medical expenses attributed to their disease, and overall medical expenses are 2.3 times higher than if they didn't have diabetes.[19] There's a lot of money to be saved by reducing or eliminating medication.

Tragically, for many, the burden of paying for the disease is overwhelming. Escalating prices are killing some of us. In 2017, Alec Smith died from insulin rationing at the age of twenty-six. He was the vanguard. More have followed because they couldn't afford their insulin and were rationing it: Jeremy Crawford, Jesimya David Scherer, Jada Renee Louis, Josh Wilkerson, Kayla Davis, Meaghan Carter, Micah Fischer, Allen Rivas, Jesse Lutgen, Alec Raeshawn Smith, Antavia Lee Worsham, Shane Patrick Boyle, and Monique Gabriel Moses.[20]

Prices have also skyrocketed in the United States. In 1996, Eli Lilly's Humalog insulin price was only twenty-one dollars for a one-month supply. By 2001, the price had increased to thirty-five dollars. In 2019, that same insulin was around $275, a 1,200 percent increase since 1996.[21] (The dollar inflated only 70 percent during the same period.) Non-insulin diabetes medications have also jumped in price. These medications are now 76 percent more expensive than they were just five years ago, driven mostly by expensive brand-name drugs such as Farxiga (dapagliflozin), Victoza, Trulicity, Januvia, and Jardiance.[22] A one-month supply of Farxiga is six hundred dollars![23] At *twenty dollars a pill*, its cost is still below other newer-generation non-insulin medications. For example, the new injectable medication mentioned previously, Wegovy, checks in at more than $1,350 per month.[24]

There's not been much competition to lower prices in the United States, although a break in this dam occurred with the late-summer 2020 introduction of Semglee by Mylan and Biocon Biologics and Walmart's offering of ReliOn brand insulin products. Semglee, a long-acting glargine insulin, is three times cheaper than the competition. ReliOn Novolog is up to 75 percent less expensive than the cash price of comparable fast-acting analog insulins. Hopefully, the trend continues.

Pushing back against pharmaceutical companies to save money isn't the answer. For starters, it's not just Big Pharma that's the problem. A complex set of supply chain members take profits, each one adding expense between the drug company and the person with diabetes. Figure 8.1 shows this tangled web for diabetes medications.

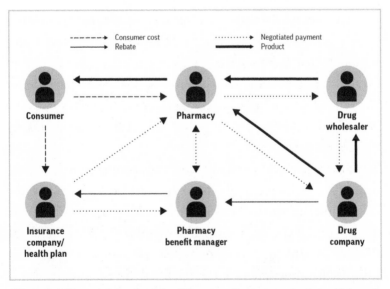

Figure 8.1. The tangled web of the diabetes medication supply chain. (Adapted from W. T. Cefalu, D. E. Dawes, G. Gavlak, et al. "Insulin Access and Affordability Working Group: Conclusions and Recommendations," *Diabetes Care* 41, no. 6 [June 2018], fig. 3.)

Everyone knows Big Pharma (e.g., Eli Lilly, Sanofi, and Novo Nordisk), but how many know the role of pharmacy benefit managers who act as middlemen between drug companies and insurers and health plans? These companies, such as Express Scripts, CVS Health, and OptumRx, have annual revenues of over $200 billion.[25] They are a significant and costly but relatively invisible part of the "multiple opaque" transactions among medication producers and channel members.[26]

Government action to break up, rein in, and otherwise detangle this supply chain web would help. An example of this can be seen in the Alec Smith Emergency Insulin Act of 2020, passed by the Minnesota state legislature, an act designed to ensure a supply of insulin in the state for those who need it to live.[27] As of spring 2020, seven states have approved copay caps on insulin purchases. The Biden administration's Build Back Better Act of 2021, not yet passed at this writing, sets copay caps at thirty-five dollars regardless of deductible. However, these government actions are just a drop in the bucket because they pertain only to insulin. And regulation such as the proposed Build Back Better Act only caps insulin *copays*, not *prices*. You still need some type of medical coverage to qualify, thus leaving the most financially vulnerable at risk.

Pharmaceutical companies could also significantly increase patient assistance programs. You know, the bit at the end of the TV commercial where the voiceover says, "If you can't afford your drugs, we might be able to help." For example, during winter 2020, Eli Lilly launched a program that allows customers to fill monthly Lilly insulin prescriptions for thirty-five dollars. However, relying on the largesse of drug companies isn't a long-term solution. (See the "Other Resources" section at the end of this chapter for links to sites that help lower costs.)

Of course, Americans could all go to Canada or Mexico for diabetes medications and get them much cheaper. But what a hassle! Or we could buy them online from these countries, but then we'd need to be careful of fake online pharmacies.* For example, 96 percent of global online pharmacies outside Canada are not trustworthy, and even 74 percent of Canadian online sites peddle medications they couldn't legally sell to Canadians—sourced from India, Turkey, or countries in Southeast Asia.[28]

Or you could practice a twelve-step perspective that leads to using a minimum of medication and relying on diet and exercise to moderate blood sugar. Those with T2D could eliminate all medications or possibly do well with just an older first-line medication like metformin, which is only two dollars a month at Walmart.[29] Those who require insulin could use much less. For example, back in the day, I cut my insulin needs by 50 percent, which reduced my diabetes medication expenses by the same percentage. This is the best way to save money. You don't have to rely on anyone but yourself, with help from your care providers, to make it happen. You'll also be much healthier.

To conclude, there's a big target on the back of Big Pharma that's easy to hit. And it should be. Diabetes medication prices and price increases in the United States are egregious. But there are other players such as pharmacy benefit managers, and much more to the story. The profit motive by itself also isn't necessarily a bad thing. Without this incentive, the

---

* For information about online pharmacy safety, see US Food and Drug Administration, "BeSafeRx: Your Source for Online Pharmacy Information," September 21, 2020, https://www.fda.gov/drugs/quick-tips-buying-medicines-over-internet/besaferx-your-source-online-pharmacy-information.

medications on which many of us rely, as well as the miracle of glucometer and continuous glucose monitoring (CGM) technology, most assuredly would not be available.

Devices

The prices of diabetes medical supplies, including devices, have stayed relatively flat in recent years, rising about 3 percent annually.[30] That's a good thing because blood glucose-monitoring technologies are crucial to living a healthy diabetes life.

Diabetes management has been transformed by glucometers and CGMs that measure blood sugar at a point in time or every five minutes, respectively. Insulin pumps have also been transformative. Glucometers and CGMs give us a blood sugar reading any time we want it. An insulin pump delivers bolus and basal insulin without injections.

Pump and CGM technologies have also been integrated to talk with one another. For example, the latest generation of pumps stops basal insulin delivery when CGM readings fall too low. This integrated technology is on the path to a true closed-loop system, otherwise known as an artificial pancreas, that perfectly controls blood sugar 24/7 without conscious effort or involvement. Pancreatic islet cells created from stem cells, which will do the same thing, are also in the works. In either case, we should be careful what we wish for.

Let's consider a person with T1D who achieves good health through a twelve-step mindset, healthy nutrition, healthy exercise, careful blood sugar monitoring, and effective dynamic diabetes management. She connects to a bona fide closed-loop artificial pancreas or gets new islet cells. After the miracle occurs, she gobbles down a chocolate sundae and has pizza for dinner. From then on, she eats the standard American diet with impunity. All the sugar, desserts, fast food, and sushi she wants!

Her future? In time, she will probably gain weight and experience insulin resistance, hyperinsulinemia, and metabolic syndrome and be on the polypharmacy path. She may develop type 2 diabetes. Her blood sugars may be in range, and hypoglycemia will be a thing of the past. But that's it. She will likely encounter health challenges that, ironically, might have been avoided if she hadn't been "cured."

Blood sugar-monitoring technology plays a significant role in safely maintaining healthy blood sugars. But it should not be used as a means of eating "normally" when doing so is just plain unhealthy. The next section outlines how these devices can and should fit in.

Dynamic Blood Sugar Management

The world-famous management consultant Peter Drucker once observed that you can't improve or manage what you can't measure. Glucometer and CGM technology have made it possible to measure (blood sugars) so those of us with diabetes can now truly dynamically improve and manage our blood sugar numbers.

Eating to the meter and Sugar Surfing are both dynamic diabetes-management tools. The former can mean checking blood sugar with a glucometer six or more times a day: before meals, two hours after, before bed, and possibly once or twice during the night. It also involves keeping a food log to track how different foods affect blood sugar. The latter elegantly uses CGM blood glucose-trend data or very frequent glucometer readings to bolus for meals and to quickly respond to blood sugar changes with insulin or carbs. *All people with diabetes can eat to the meter.* Sugar Surfing, however, is appropriate only for those who manage diabetes with mealtime bolus and basal insulin.

EATING TO THE METER

It has been possible to dynamically manage blood sugar since glucometer technology arrived in the early 1980s. Before then, a person with T2D might take an unchanging regimen of medication—let's say metformin in the morning and a long-acting insulin at night. He or she might eat the standard American diet, not exercise much, and suffer poor health.

With eating to the meter, people with type 2 stay with the same medication routine *but only as a starting point.* From there, through regular glucometer checks, the person with T2D eats and exercises healthily while maintaining a daily logbook to learn the effects that their healthy diet has on blood sugar. They learn from experience what different foods do to their blood sugars, including foods to avoid even within the context of a healthy diet, and how to smooth out glycemic spikes. Blood sugar management goes from static and passive to dynamic and active.

If a glucometer reading is elevated before a meal, a person with T2D might eat fewer, if any, carbs for that meal. They might even go on a brisk twenty-minute walk after lunch to lower their blood sugar. Since they have already embarked on a healthier way of eating and exercising based on the principles covered in this book, these dynamic practices make an improved situation even better.

This person eats to the meter day in and day out with glucometer checks before *every* meal and a check two hours after a meal. They also do a check at bedtime and in the middle of the night. In time, A1c levels drop to a normal range for people in general, not just "good enough" for people with diabetes.

The diet logbook may eventually be put away as this person learns the effects of exercise and healthy food and stays firmly on their dietary plank. As health improves, the person may be able to cut back on glucometer checks to premeal only and ideally, with the assistance of their care provider, eliminate medication. If this occurs, blood sugar checks might be reduced to perhaps just a few per week, or under special circumstances such as an illness or before a medical procedure.

Those who rely on insulin can also eat to the meter. Static bolus and correction insulin ratios then become *starting points* for dynamic management as described above, not the only option. For example, based on premeal blood sugar levels, a person with T1D might increase bolus insulin. Or, based on the prospect of vigorous exercise and a glucometer reading, turn off the basal rate on their pump or eat glucose. A correction bolus might be less than a predetermined amount because of the time of day and the person's knowledge of their blood sugars at that particular time. It's a coincidence if, on any two days, the person with T1D uses the same amount of insulin. The primary drag to eating to the meter for an insulin-dependent person is that they can't eventually put away the meter. Blood sugar still needs to be tested five or more times each day.

SUGAR SURFING

Sugar Surfing™ represents the next level of dynamic diabetes management. It was created by Dr. Stephen Ponder and Kevin McMahon and is intended for those who depend on bolus and basal insulin.[31] Rather than eating to the meter based on only five or six glucometer readings a day, a sugar surfer recognizes and responds to blood sugar patterns using CGM readings (one every five minutes) or data from a flash monitoring system, such as a FreeStyle Libre.

The surfer continually rides the glycemic wave, anticipating trends, dosing boluses, and continuously correcting with "nudges" of insulin and carbs. Static insulin bolus and correction ratios are still in play, but *only as starting points* for daily glycemic-wave-riding. Figure 8.2 outlines the process and basic principles of Sugar Surfing.

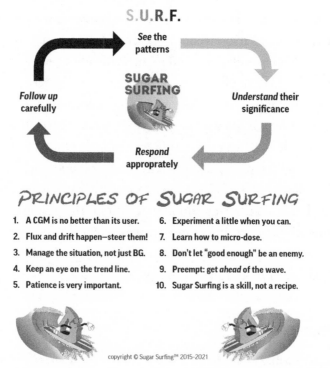

Figure 8.2. The process and principles of Sugar Surfing™. (Reprinted by permission of Stephen W. Ponder and Kevin L. McMahon [sugarsurfing.com].)

Sugar Surfing does not require insulin infused from a pump. Multidose insulin therapy (MDI) with a pen or syringe works fine. Following the six rules of healthy diabetic eating while sitting on either plank on the diabetes teeter-totter works great, although lower-carb or ketogenic eating is more manageable.[†]

I'd been Sugar Surfing for years before I even knew the term. It would have been difficult for me or anyone else to precisely define or teach how to do it. Dr. Ponder and Mr. McMahon have filled this gap. Sugar Surfing is a skill that needs to be learned, and it's worth the effort. The best way to start is by reading the book *Sugar Surfing* listed at the end of this chapter. It's available through the usual online outlets or at sugarsurfing.com.

We're in the home stretch! The next chapter briefly puts everything together with some caveats.

Dr. Randy Elde Weighs In on Drugs and Devices

As a practicing pharmacist for over forty years and a diabetes care and education specialist for twenty-four years, I have witnessed an explosion of medication use in our country such that today the United States now has one of the

continued

---

† I've seen Dr. Ponder demonstrate the efficacy of Sugar Surfing using the example of a cheeseburger and onion rings. I don't recommend this for the many reasons covered in this book, but it is occasionally possible for a skilled surfer.

highest medication-use rates per capita in the world. (As noted in the chapter, this phenomenon is labeled polypharmacy.) Certainly, medical conditions like heart disease and diabetes may require multiple medications, but reducing the number of them taken is best for patients for the reasons Chad has listed.

Multiple studies have demonstrated that the simpler any medication regimen is, the more likely it will be followed. If a patient is to take one tablet per day, they are highly likely to do so—but more frequent dosing is less likely to be adhered to. Prescribing the appropriate medication is always important, but sometimes deprescribing or discontinuing a medication that is no longer needed is just as important.

Both the American Diabetes Association and the American Association of Clinical Endocrinologists produce updated guidance each year on all aspects of diabetes care. These are the principal guidelines that providers use to direct their care. For several years now, both sets of guidelines have extolled the primary importance of lifestyle changes, but this needs even more emphasis—because all too often the recommendation is disregarded in favor of prescription medications. In short, whenever possible, it's usually best for you and your care provider to think in terms of nutrition and exercise first and then consider medications.

Again, this is not to minimize the importance of needed medications; for example, many cannot do without insulin.

An often-overlooked method for evaluating one's medication list is to turn to a personal pharmacist for expertise.

Many insurance plans, including Medicare, will pay for a periodic extensive consultation with a pharmacist, referred to as medication therapy management. This consultation will examine your entire medication regimen, including analyzing the appropriateness of each drug for you, potential side effects, potential interactions, cost-saving options, whether the medications are being used correctly, and any duplication of medications.

During such reviews, on several occasions, I uncovered a patient's misunderstanding of their insulin. Many insulin-requiring patients use two different types: mealtime insulin and longer-acting basal insulin. In one instance, a patient was using two mealtime insulins, and on another occasion, a patient was using two long-acting insulins. In both cases, their blood sugar control was inadequate and, at times, in danger of leading to significantly low blood sugar reactions.

It's important to be aware of any medication side effects, including the relative incidence of any effect. Does the side effect occur in a significant number of patients, or is the incidence so low that you're very unlikely to experience the effect? It's also important to recognize that the side effect profile of a drug can change over time. As continued experience occurs with any drug, additional side effects may be noted, or previously mentioned significant side effects may turn out to be of minimal significance. This is similarly true with drug interactions: What is the significance of a potential interaction? Your pharmacist is a wonderful resource to help sort out this information for you.

continued

Unfortunately, many patients with diabetes have other medical conditions such as high blood pressure or high cholesterol. Some of the medications used to treat these conditions are also involved in the most commonly seen drug interactions. On one such occasion, a patient of mine was experiencing considerable side effects from his cholesterol medicine. He had been taking it for several years without any noticeable problems. I learned that he had recently started a new blood pressure medicine, which was around the same time the side effect began. My investigation revealed that the new blood pressure medicine increased levels of the cholesterol medication, which in turn caused discomfort. Through discussions with his care provider, the patient was able to reduce the dose of his cholesterol medication. My follow-up revealed no deterioration in the patient's cholesterol lab values, and his side effect disappeared.

The price we pay for drugs in the United States is receiving more—and needed—attention, especially the cost of insulin. The complexity of this issue, coupled with political stalemates in our country, leads to feelings of helplessness for many. Again, focusing on nutrition and exercise can empower people with greater agency.

*   *   *

Dr. Randy Elde, a retired certified diabetes care and education specialist, earned his doctorate in pharmacy in 2011 and became board-certified in advanced diabetes management in 2014. Dr. Elde's involvement in diabetes care was piqued nearly thirty years ago by his daughter's diagnosis of type 1 diabetes in her adolescence. His career in western Washington State as a pharmacist and diabetes educator spanned over forty years. In 2017, the Washington Association of Diabetes Educators honored him with their Diabetes Educator of the Year award.

Whether in pharmacy or diabetes care, his driving force was the personal relationships he established with patients, in which he strove to always be the best listener. In addition to his daughter, he credits all the young children with diabetes with whom he was honored to work with for many years as part of the medical staff at a summer camp for these children.

Questions for Your Care Providers

Several of the following questions can also be addressed by Dr. Elde's suggestion that you seek out a medication therapy management session with your local pharmacist. You might even consider doing this to get a second option.

- *What are the effects of my medication(s)? Why have I been prescribed them?*

- *What is the process for managing their dosages? How frequently should dosages be reviewed?* It may be time to revisit Chapter 4's questions for your care provider that deal with staging reduction in medication as your health improves.

- *What are the side effects of my medications? What should I look out for?*

- *Do my medications interact? If so, with what and at what level (minor, moderate, major)? What should I look out for?*

- *Are there side effects or interactions associated with the supplements I'm taking?* Nonprescription supplements and vitamins also need to be part of this conversation!

- *Are there generic or less costly options for my medications, medical supplies, and devices?*

- *What are your views of dynamic diabetes management?* This question offers the opportunity for a more wide-ranging conversation about the process of managing diabetes.

Further Reading

BOOKS

- Dubois, Wil. *Beyond Fingersticks: The Art of Control with Continuous Glucose Monitoring.* Las Vegas, NM: Red Blood Cell Books, 2010. (Though Wil published this CGM book more than ten years ago, it still provides an excellent overview.)

- Ponder, Stephen W., and Kevin L. McMahon. *Sugar Surfing: How to Manage Type 1 Diabetes in a Modern World.* Sausalito, CA: Mediself Press, 2015.

- Scheiner, Gary. *Think Like a Pancreas: A Practical Guide to Managing Diabetes with Insulin.* 3rd ed. New York:

Hachette, 2020. (A superb reference for those of us who are insulin-dependent.)

OTHER RESOURCES

- Behring, S. "16 Tips to Help You Afford Your Diabetes Medication and Supplies." *Healthline*, May 3, 2021. https://www.healthline.com/health/diabetes/16-tips-to -help-you-afford-your-diabetes-medication-and-supplies.

- Dubois, Wil. "Your Ultimate Guide to Glucose Monitoring." *Diabetes Self-Management*, Winter 2021. https://www.scribd.com/article/536501044/ Your-Ultimate-Guide-To-Glucose-Monitoring.

- GoodRx: goodrx.com. This is an excellent source for prescription drug costs and availability.

- JDRF. "Help with Your Diabetes Prescription and Insulin Costs." https://www.jdrf.org/t1d-resources/living-with -t1d/insurance/help-with-prescription-costs. (A site to check for lower prices for all diabetes medications.)

- WebMD and Medscape: webmd.com and medscape.com/ today. These are good places to check out prescription drug side effects and interactions.

CHAPTER 9

PUTTING IT ALL TOGETHER

My research, writing, consulting, and teaching through the years have revolved around management philosophy and practice. Consequently, it's not surprising that I view management, as in dynamic diabetes management, as the key to doing diabetes differently and better. After all, a carpenter with a hammer sees every problem as a nail! Still, Figure 9.1, a graphic that ties all parts of the book together, makes a convincing case for dynamic diabetes management as the lynchpin to good health.

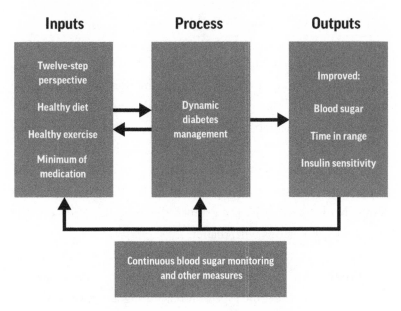

Figure 9.1. Empowering a healthier you.

The inputs of adapting and applying a twelve-step perspective to living with diabetes (Chapters 3 and 4); healthy diet and exercise (Chapters 5, 6, and 7), and using a minimum of medication (Chapter 8), when dynamically and effectively managed (the process, Chapter 8), leads to positive outputs of improved blood sugars, time in range, and insulin sensitivity. Numbers from continuous blood sugar monitoring and other measures such as A1cs, GlycoMark (a measure of the extent of recent hyperglycemic events), cholesterol and triglycerides, weight gain or loss, and CGM or glucometer reports make continuous improvement possible and drive the entire system.

All systems, such as the one depicted in Figure 9.1, tend to be only as strong as their weakest link. Your inputs could be spot-on. You are positioned to use a minimum of medication through healthy eating and exercise, but poor management leads to problems. For example, your blood sugar isn't monitored continuously, so you can't effectively manage blood sugar changes. Conversely, you could do a great job of dynamic management. But poor eating and exercise sabotage the process. It's tough to manage a blood sugar spike dynamically and effectively after consuming a cheeseburger, onion rings, and a caramel milkshake. All parts of a system need to work well together.

Maintaining a daily routine is also important to the successful practice of the system depicted in Figure 9.1 in real life. Riva Greenberg describes its importance this way, a description that applies to all persons with diabetes:

> Routine, for me is a major tool managing my blood glucose: eating the same type of foods, eating about the same time of day, walking an hour a day usually at the same time, checking my blood glucose frequently. . . . I'm disciplined, pay attention, do the work, and the regularity of routine reduces the fluxes of unpredictability.[1]

I wrap up with some closing thoughts. First, my ideas don't apply to all of us. Dynamic diabetes management is much easier to adopt for the affluent than for the poor. Many can't afford to eat healthily or buy medical supplies. Food deserts in America mean quality food isn't available even if people could buy it. Glucometer test strips and CGM supplies are expensive. Those living in food deserts are many of the same people who have trouble affording basic diabetes medication, much less three hundred dollars for a one-month supply of CGM sensors or five dollars a day for test strips. They may have little or no insurance. That's not right.

Second, I have written this book for adults, not kids. By themselves, young children will not understand or may not have the capability to adopt all of the mindset, nutritional, exercise, and diabetes management principles and practices outlined in this book. Plus, I wouldn't want my six-year-old to have to say no to cake at a birthday party.

An adult with a twelve-step perspective can more comfortably decline the cake at the same birthday party or eat a salad while his friends chow down on pizza. It's just a different situation with kids and even teenagers. Still, much is possible with the close support of family. For example, Dr. Ponder has taught children to sugar surf. Dr. Bernstein has helped parents of children with T1D learn healthy ketogenic eating.[2] Jeff Hitchcock's excellent book for parents of diabetic kids is listed in the "Further Reading" section at the end of this chapter. (A link to Mr. Hitchcock's Children with Diabetes organization is also listed at the end of this chapter. This organization has done terrific work with diabetic children and their families.)

You may have care providers who are unwilling or unable to answer your questions, lack the time, or are otherwise bound to outdated practices. A shortage of endocrinologists in the United States doesn't make this situation any easier. Hopefully, this book has still helped you to frame questions in your search for answers from qualified care providers.

To close, you don't have to accept diabetes as a progressive condition. You don't have to accept falling apart and dying young. It is possible to safely maintain healthy blood sugars using much less medication. It is possible to live a long and healthy life.

I wish you well.

Questions for Your Care Providers

- *What are two or three of the best ways to slow down or to stop the progression of my diabetes?* This is a catch-all question intended to help you and your care provider to prioritize the next best steps for your care.

- *How might we best work together to coordinate all parts of my care, including the mental part, nutrition, exercise, and drugs and devices?*

Further Reading

- Children with Diabetes: childrenwithdiabetes.com

- Hitchcock, Jeff. *101 Tips for Parents of Kids with Diabetes.* New York, NY: Skyhorse, 2016.

ACKNOWLEDGMENTS

I thank all who provided expert commentaries: Riva Greenberg (diabetes and its treatment), Ginger Vieira (the mental part), Dr. Jody Stanislaw (nutrition), Delaine Wright (exercise), and Dr. Randy Elde (drugs and devices).

Thanks especially go to Randy, a DCES and PharmD, and to Laird Findlay, MD and internist, who met regularly with me to fact-check, talk, and drink coffee. Other fact-checkers and reviewers to whom I give thanks include clinical nutritionist Karl Mincin; diabetes medical writer Carol Verderese; endocrinologists Drs. Stephen Ponder and Irl Hirsch; Jeff Hitchcock, founder of Children with Diabetes; Wil Dubois, diabetes author, educator, columnist, and blogger; and Amber Clour, cofounder and host of *Diabetes Daily Grind* and *Real Life Diabetes Podcast*.

Wil also served as an editor, along with Mi Ae Lipe. Both did a fabulous job of proofing every word. Appreciation also goes to my brother, Phil, for his word-processing fixes. Boudewijn Bertsch, codeveloper of the Flourishing Treatment Approach

(FTA) in diabetes, saved the day for me with his help on the book title. I also thank once again Bou's partner in FTA (and life), Riva Greenberg, for her excellent recommendations. A special thank-you goes to literary agent Linda Konner. Linda went above and beyond to help me to understand the nuances and challenges of traditional publishing.

The Greenleaf Book Group people who worked on the production and marketing of my book earn a special thank-you. Rebecca Logan and Claudia Volkman made a good book much better.

I dedicate this book to Drs. Laird Findlay, Richard Bernstein, and Irl Hirsch, and to my wife, Patty. Laird became a friend as my family doctor of almost forty years. He guided my earlier diabetes journey with compassion and competence. I've never met Dr. Bernstein, but his book opened my eyes. Dr. Hirsch has been my endocrinologist for the past ten years. His encyclopedic understanding kept me from falling over a cliff and constructively grounded me when we discussed this book. These physicians and Patty saved my life. I can't thank them enough.

Patricia, my wife of forty-four years, was a caregiver before I met the others. She has saved me in more ways than one. Those living with an insulin-dependent person can appreciate the challenges of day-to-day life with us, such as the time I threw orange juice in Patty's face or the many times I almost died. There are now far fewer challenges, thanks to the contributions of Drs. Findlay, Bernstein, and Hirsch. Patty thanks them also.

NOTES

CHAPTER 1

1. I. B. Hirsch, "Glycemic Variability and Diabetes Complications: Does It Matter? Of Course It Does!" *Diabetes Care* 38, no. 8 (August 2015): 1610–1614.

2. R. D. Feinman, W. K. Pogozelski, A. Astrup, R. K. Bernstein, E. J. Fine, E. C. Westman, A. Accurso, et al., "Dietary Carbohydrate Restriction as the First Approach in Diabetes Management: Critical Review and Evidence Base," *Nutrition* 31, no. 1 (January 2015): 1–13.

3. E. A. Sims, E. Danforth Jr., E. S. Horton, G. A. Bray, J. A. Glennon, and L. B. Salans, "Endocrine and Metabolic Effects of Experimental Obesity in Man," *Recent Progress in Hormone Research* 29 (1973): 457–496.

4. A. Powell, "Obesity? Diabetes? We've Been Set Up," *Harvard Gazette*, March 7, 2012, https://news.harvard.edu/gazette/story/2012/03/the-big-setup/.

5. J. Fung, *The Diabetes Code: Prevent and Reverse Type 2 Diabetes Naturally* (Vancouver: Greystone Books, 2018).

6. A. Tanzi, "The Average American Is Edging Closer to Being Borderline Obese," *Bloomberg*, December 20, 2018, https://www.bloombergquint.com/onweb/tale-of-the-tape-average-american-is-borderline-obese-cdc-says.

7. D. Hurley, *Diabetes Rising: How a Rare Disease Became a Modern Pandemic, and What to Do about It* (New York: Kaplan, 2011).

8. L. J. Andes, Y. J. Cheng, D. B. Rolka, E. W. Gregg, and G. Imperatore, "Prevalence of Prediabetes among Adolescents and Young Adults in the United States, 2005–2016," *JAMA Pediatrics* 174, no. 2 (February 2020): e194498, doi:10.1001/jamapediatrics.2019.4498.

9. E. Ahlqvist, P. Storm, A. Käräjämäki, M. Martinell, M. Dorkhan, A. Carlsson, P. Vikman, et al., "Novel Subgroups of Adult-Onset Diabetes and Their Association with Outcomes: A Data-Driven Cluster Analysis of Six Variables," *Lancet* 6, no. 5 (May 2018): 361–369.

10. Centers for Disease Control and Prevention, *National Diabetes Statistics Report, 2020: Estimates of Diabetes and Its Burden in the United States* (Atlanta, GA: Centers for Disease Control and Prevention, 2020).

11. A. G. Tabák, C. Herder, W. Rathmann, E. J. Brunner, and M. Kivimäki, "Prediabetes: A High-Risk State for Diabetes Development," *Lancet* 379, no. 9833 (2012): 2279–2290.

12. Centers for Disease Control and Prevention, *National Diabetes Statistics Report, 2020.*

13. American Diabetes Association, "Economic Costs of Diabetes in the U.S. in 2017," *Diabetes Care* 41, no. 5 (May 2018): 917–928.

14. Ibid.

15. National Institutes of Health, "Estimates of Funding for Various Research, Condition, and Disease Categories (RCDC)," February 24, 2020, https://report.nih.gov/categorical_spending.aspx.

CHAPTER 2

1. W. Davis, *Undoctored: Why Health Care Has Failed You and How You Can Become Smarter Than Your Doctor* (New York: Rodale Books, 2017), ix.

2. S. V. Edelman (and Friends), *Taking Control of Your Diabetes*, 4th ed. (West Islip, NY: Professional Communications, 2012).

3. K. M. Adams, M. Kohlmeier, and S. H. Zeisel, "Nutrition Education in U.S. Medical Schools: Latest Update of a National Survey," *Academic Medicine* 85, no. 9 (September 2010): 1537–1542.

4. S. Devries, A. Agatston, M. Aggarwal, K. E. Aspry, C. B. Esselstyn, P. Kris-Etherton, M. Miller, et al., "A Deficiency of Nutrition Education and Practice in Cardiology," *American Journal of Medicine* 130, no. 11 (November 2017): 1298–1305.

5. Deloitte Center for Health Solutions, "Deloitte 2012 Survey of U.S. Health Care Consumers: The Performance of the Health Care System and Health Care Reform," 2012, https://www2.deloitte.com/content/dam/Deloitte/us/Documents/life-sciences-health-care/us-lshc-2012-survey-of-us-consumers-health-care.pdf.

6. R. Greenberg and B. Bertsch, "The Flourishing Treatment Approach: A Strengths-Based Model Informed by How People Create Health," *Diabetes Care and Education* 37, no. 6 (December 2016): 39–44.

7. S. Perrine, "7 Heart Numbers That May Reveal Health Risks," *AARP*, February 8, 2019, https://www.aarp.org/health/conditions-treatments/info-2019/7-heart-health-numbers.html#quest1.

8. J. Bardsley, "What Happens When MyPlate Sets the Menu? A Starch Overload," *Daily Herald*, September 1, 2019, https://www.heraldnet.com/life/what-happens-when-myplate-sets-the-menu-a-starch-overload/.

9. American Diabetes Association, "Recipes and Nutrition: Eat Good to Feel Good," accessed April 28, 2022, https://diabetes.org/healthy-living/recipes-nutrition/eating-well.

10. H. Warshaw, "Diabetes Management and Nutrition Guide: ADA's 2019 Nutrition Therapy Consensus Report," *Today's Dietician*, July 2019, https://www.todaysdietitian.com/newarchives/0719p36.shtml.

11. R. Minners, "Living History," *Diabetes Forecast*, November–December 2015, https://www.slideshare.net/ReganWrightMinners/adatimeline.

12. G. L. King, *Reverse Your Diabetes in 12 Weeks: The Scientifically Proven Program to Avoid, Control, and Turn Around Your Diabetes* (New York: Workman, 2016).

13. R. K. Bernstein, *Dr. Bernstein's Diabetes Solution: The Complete Guide to Achieving Normal Blood Sugars*, 4th ed. (New York: Little, Brown Spark, 2011).

14. L. Fisher, J. S. Gonzalez, and W. H. Polonsky, "The Confusing Tale of Depression and Distress in Patients with Diabetes: A Call for Greater Clarity and Precision," *Diabetic Medicine* 31, no. 7 (July 2014): 764–772.

15. Diabetes Psychologist, "The Ultimate Guide to Getting Unstuck with T1D," accessed April 28, 2022, https://www.thediabetespsychologist .com/get-unstuck-free-download.

16. N. Saunders, "Your No-Burnout, Manage-It-All Plan," *Living Well with Diabetes*, September 2018.

17. Greenberg and Bertsch, "The Flourishing Treatment Approach."

18. R. Greenberg and B. Bertsch, "When Disease Requires a Complexity Framework," in *Cynefin: Weaving Sense-Making into the Fabric of Our World*, ed. Riva Greenberg and Boudewijn Bertsch (Singapore: Cognitive Edge, 2021), 153–168.

CHAPTER 3

1. V. H. Vroom, *Work and Motivation* (New York: Wiley, 1964).

2. D. M. Nathan, "The Diabetes Control and Complications Trial/ Epidemiology of Diabetes Interventions and Complications Study at 30 Years: Overview," *Diabetes Care* 37, no. 1 (January 2014): 9–16.

3. A. Brown, *Bright Spots and Landmines: The Diabetes Guide I Wish Someone Had Handed Me* (San Francisco: diaTribe Foundation, 2017). Adam Brown has published an update to the book: see A. Brown, "42 Factors That Affect Blood Glucose?! A Surprising Update," *DiaTribe Learn*, February 13, 2018, https://diatribe.org/42factors.

4. S. E. Richards, "Your Sugar Playbook," *Living Well with Diabetes*, September 2018, p. 40.

5. "Five Diabetes Diet Myths," *Outsmart Diabetes*, 2015.

6. A. Tsai, "What's Your Diabetes IQ?" *Diabetes Forecast*, May 2018.

7. M. Lenoir, F. Serre, L. Cantin, and S. H. Ahmed, "Intense Sweetness Surpasses Cocaine Reward," *PLoS ONE* 2, no. 8 (August 2007): e698, doi.org/10.1371/journal.pone.0000698.

8. D. M. Blumenthal and M. S. Gold, "Neurobiology of Food Addiction," *Current Opinion in Clinical Nutrition and Metabolic Care* 13, no. 4 (July 2010): 359–365.

9. S. J. Guyenet, "Why Are Some People 'Carboholics'?" *Science of Body Weight and Health* (blog), July 26, 2017, https://www.stephanguyenet .com/why-are-some-people-carboholics/.

10. SugarScience, "How Much Is Too Much?" accessed June 18, 2020, https://sugarscience.ucsf.edu/dispelling-myths-too-much.html# .YmtvqpPMI4i.

11. C. D. Fryar, J. P. Hughes, K. A. Herrick, and N. Ahluwalia, "Fast Food Consumption among Adults in the United States, 2013–2016," *NCHS Data Brief*, no. 322 (October 2018): 1–8.

12. "Share-Worthy Diabetes Life Hacks," *DiabetesMine*, April 18, 2019, https://www.healthline.com/diabetesmine/diabetes-life-hacks.

13. G. Scheiner, "My Diabetes Confession," Integrated Diabetes Services, March 21, 2014, https://integrateddiabetes.com/ my-diabetes-confession/.

14. J. K. Dickinson, "Retire Negative Language Associated with Diabetes," *Diabetes Forecast*, March 2018.

CHAPTER 4

1. G. Taubes, *Good Calories, Bad Calories: Fats, Carbs, and the Controversial Science of Diet and Health* (New York: Anchor Books, 2008).

2. R. R. Henry, B. Gumbiner, T. Ditzler, P. Wallace, R. Lyon, and H. S. Glauber, "Intensive Conventional Insulin Therapy for Type II Diabetes: Metabolic Effects during a 6-Mo Outpatient Trial," *Diabetes Care* 16, no. 1 (January 1993): 21–31.

3. P. A. Velasquez-Mieyer, P. A. Cowan, K. L. Arheart, C. K. Buffington, K. A. Spencer, B. E. Connelly, G. W. Cowan, and R. H. Lustig, "Suppression of Insulin Secretion Is Associated with Weight Loss and Altered Macronutrient Intake and Preference in a Subset of Obese Adults," *International Journal of Obesity* 27, no. 2 (February 2003): 219–226.

4. "The U.S. Weight Loss Market in 2018—Forecasts," *Webwire*, December 6, 2017, https://www.webwire.com/ViewPressRel .asp?aId=217481.

5. Jenny Craig, "Plans and Pricing," accessed September 6, 2020, https:// www.jennycraig.com/shop-plans.

6. D. Pollock, *You Can Achieve Normal Blood Sugar: Discover the Surprising Results from Over 100 Blood Sugar Tests* (Eugene, OR: Harvest House, 2019).

7. J. Fritsch, "95% Regain Lost Weight: Or Do They?" *New York Times*, May 25, 1999, https://www.nytimes.com/1999/05/25/health/95 -regain-lost-weight-or-do-they.html.

8. J. C. Kerns, J. Guo, E. Fothergill, L. Howard, N. D. Knuth, R. Brychta, K. Y. Chen, et al., "Increased Physical Activity Associated with Less Weight Regain Six Years after 'The Biggest Loser' Competition," *Obesity* 25, no. 11 (November 2017): 1838–1843.

9. E. Loveman, G. K. Frampton, J. Shepherd, J. Picot, K. Cooper, J. Bryant, K. Welch, and A. Clegg, "The Clinical Effectiveness and Cost-Effectiveness of Long-Term Weight Management Schemes for Adults: A Systematic Review," *Health Technology Assessment* 15, no. 2 (January 2011): 1–182.

10. M. J. Franz, J. L. Boucher, S. Rutten-Ramos, and J. J. VanWormer, "Lifestyle Weight-Loss Intervention Outcomes in Overweight and Obese Adults with Type 2 Diabetes: A Systematic Review and Meta-analysis of Randomized Clinical Trials," *Journal of the Academy of Nutrition and Dietetics* 115, no. 9 (September 2015): 1447–1463.

11. M. G. Salvia, "The Look AHEAD Trial: Translating Lessons Learned into Clinical Practice and Further Study," *Diabetes Spectrum* 30, no. 3 (August 2017): 166–170.

12. T. J. Graham, D. S. Bond, S. Phelan, J. O. Hill, and R. R. Wing, "Weight-Loss Maintenance for 10 Years in the National Weight Control Registry," *American Journal of Preventive Medicine* 46, no. 1 (January 2014): 17–23.

13. National Weight Control Registry, "NWCR Facts," accessed June 18, 2020, http://nwcr.ws/Research/default.htm; H. A. Raynor, R. W. Jeffery, S. Phelan, J. O. Hill, and R. R. Wing, "Amount of Food

Group Variety Consumed in the Diet and Long-Term Weight Loss Maintenance," *Obesity Research* 13, no. 5 (May 2005): 883–890.

14. L. W. Hill and R. S. Eckman, *The Starvation Treatment of Diabetes, with a Series of Graduated Diets* (Boston: W. M. Leonard, 1917).

15. T. T. Gorski and M. Miller, *Staying Sober: A Guide for Relapse Prevention* (Independence, MO: Herald House/Independence Press, 2013).

16. Alcoholics Anonymous, "2014 Membership Survey," 2014, https://www.aa.org/sites/default/files/literature/assets/p-48_membershipsurvey.pdf; L. Dodes and Z. Dodes, *The Sober Truth: Debunking the Bad Science Behind 12-Step Programs and the Rehab Industry* (Boston: Beacon Press, 2014); R. H. Moos and B. S. Moos, "Participation in Treatment and Alcoholics Anonymous: A 16-Year Follow-Up of Initially Untreated Individuals," *Journal of Clinical Psychology* 62, no. 6 (June 2006): 735–750.

17. Quoted in Bruce Thomas, *Bruce Lee: Fighting Spirit* (Berkeley, CA: Frog, 1994), 44.

CHAPTER 5

1. K. Close and A. Brown, "CGM and Time-in-Range: What Do Diabetes Experts Think about Goals?" DiaTribe Learn, December 20, 2017, https://diatribe.org/cgm-and-time-range-what-do-diabetes-experts-think-about-goals.

2. J. A. McDougall, "Diabetes (Adult Onset and Juvenile)," Dr. McDougall's Health and Medical Center, accessed June 18, 2020, https://www.drmcdougall.com/health/education/health-science/common-health-problems/diabetes-adult-onset-and-juvenile/.

3. N. D. Barnard, *Dr. Neal Barnard's Program for Reversing Diabetes* (Emmaus, PA: Rodale Books, 2006).

4. J. Fung, *The Diabetes Code: Prevent and Reverse Type 2 Diabetes Naturally* (Vancouver: Greystone Books, 2018).

5. A. J. Garber, M. J. Abrahamson, J. I. Barzilay, L. Blonde, Z. T. Bloomgarden, M. A. Bush, S. Dagogo-Jack, et al., "Consensus Statement by the American Association of Clinical Endocrinologists and American College of Endocrinology on the Comprehensive

Type 2 Diabetes Management Algorithm: 2019 Executive Summary," *Endocrine Practice* 25, no. 1 (January 2019): 69–100.

6. I. M. Stratton, A. I. Adler, H. A. Neil, D. R. Matthews, S. E. Manley, C. A. Cull, D. Hadden, R. C. Turner, and R. R. Holman, "Association of Glycaemia with Macrovascular and Microvascular Complications of Type 2 Diabetes (UKPDS 35): Prospective Observational Study," *BMJ* 321 (August 2000): 405–412.

7. J.-P. Després, B. Lamarche, P. Mauriège, B. Cantin, G. R. Dagenais, S. Moorjani, and P. J. Lupien, "Hyperinsulinemia as an Independent Risk Factor for Ischemic Heart Disease," *New England Journal of Medicine* 334, no. 15 (April 1996): 952–958; J.-M. Gamble, S. H. Simpson, D. T. Eurich, S. R. Majumdar, and J. A. Johnson, "Insulin Use and Increased Risk of Mortality in Type 2 Diabetes: A Cohort Study," *Diabetes, Obesity and Metabolism* 12, no. 1 (January 2010): 47–53.

8. R. K. Bernstein, *Dr. Bernstein's Diabetes Solution: The Complete Guide to Achieving Normal Blood Sugars*, 4th ed. (New York: Little, Brown Spark, 2011).

9. R. G. Dluhy and G. T. McMahon, "Intensive Glycemic Control in the ACCORD and ADVANCE Trials," *New England Journal of Medicine* 358, no. 24 (June 2008): 2630–2633.

10. I. B. Hirsch, J. L. Sherr, and K. K. Hood, "Connecting the Dots: Validation of Time in Range Metrics with Microvascular Outcomes," *Diabetes Care* 42, no. 3 (March 2019): 345–348.

11. L. A. C. Wright and I. B. Hirsch, "Metrics beyond Hemoglobin A1C in Diabetes Management: Time in Range, Hypoglycemia, and Other Parameters," *Diabetes Technology and Therapeutics* 19, no. S2 (May 2017): S16–S26.

12. Bernstein, *Dr. Bernstein's Diabetes Solution.*

13. C. D. Fryar, J. P. Hughes, K. A. Herrick, and N. Ahluwalia, "Fast Food Consumption among Adults in the United States, 2013–2016," *NCHS Data Brief*, no. 322 (October 2018): 1–8.

14. O. Ahern, P. M. Gatcomb, N. A. Held, W. A. Petit Jr., and W. V. Tamborlane, "Exaggerated Hyperglycemia after a Pizza Meal in Well-Controlled Diabetes," *Diabetes Care* 16, no. 4 (April 1993): 578–580.

15. J. Ruhl, "Calculate Your Ideal Nutrient Intake for Weight Loss or Maintenance," accessed June 18, 2020, http://jennybrown.net/Calculators/DietMakeupCalcNew.htm.

16. M. A. Paterson, B. R. King, C. E. M. Smart, T. Smith, J. Rafferty, and P. E. Lopez, "Impact of Dietary Protein on Postprandial Glycaemic Control and Insulin Requirements in Type 1 Diabetes: A Systematic Review," *Diabetic Medicine* 36, no. 12 (2019): 1585–1599.

17. V. Stefansson, "Food and Food Habits in Alaska and Northern Canada," in *Human Nutrition: Historic and Scientific*, ed. I. Galdston (New York: International Universities Press, 1960), 23–60.

18. V. Stefansson, "Adventures in Diet, Part 2," *Harper's Monthly Magazine*, December 1935, https://biblelife.org/stefansson2.htm.

19. A. Ewbank, "The Arctic Explorer Who Pushed an All-Meat Diet," *Atlas Obscura*, August 28, 2018, https://www.atlasobscura.com/articles/all-meat-diet.

20. E. Davis and K. Runyan, *The Ketogenic Diet for Type 1 Diabetes: Reduce Your HbA1c and Avoid Diabetic Complications* (Cheyenne, WY: Gutsy Badger, 2017).

21. J. Bowden, *Living Low Carb: Controlled-Carbohydrate Eating for Long-Term Weight Loss* (New York: Sterling, 2013).

22. G. Taubes, *Good Calories, Bad Calories: Fats, Carbs, and the Controversial Science of Diet and Health* (New York: Anchor Books, 2008).

23. R. J. de Souza, A. Mente, A. Maroleanu, A. I. Cozma, V. Ha, T. Kishibi, E. Uleryk, et al., "Intake of Saturated and Trans Unsaturated Fatty Acids and Risk of All-Cause Mortality, Cardiovascular Disease, and Type 2 Diabetes: Systematic Review and Meta-analysis of Observational Studies," *BMJ* 351 (August 2015): h3978, https://doi.org/10.1136/bmj.h3978; P. W. Siri-Tarino, Q. Sun, F. B. Hu, and R. M. Krauss, "Meta-analysis of Prospective Cohort Studies Evaluating the Association of Saturated Fat with Cardiovascular Disease," *American Journal of Clinical Nutrition* 91, no. 3 (March 2010): 535–546.

24. U. Ravnskov, M. de Lorgeril, D. M. Diamond, R. Hama, T. Hamazaki, B. Hammarskjold, N. Hynes, et al., "LDL-C Does Not Cause Cardiovascular Disease: A Comprehensive Review of the Current Literature," *Expert Review of Clinical Pharmacology* 11, no. 10 (October

2018): 959–970; R. DuBroff and M. de Lorgeril, "Cholesterol Confusion and Statin Controversy," *World Journal of Cardiology* 7, no. 7 (July 2015): 404–409.

25.   B. Bale, and A. Doneen, *Beat the Heart Attack Gene: The Revolutionary Plan to Prevent Heart Disease, Stroke, and Diabetes* (New York: Wiley, 2014).

26.   R. Roberts, "Genetics of Coronary Artery Disease: An Update," *Methodist DeBakey Cardiovascular Journal* 10, no. 1 (January–March 2014): 7–12.

27.   A. Sachdeva, C. P. Cannon, P. C. Deedwania, K. A. Labresh, S. C. Smith Jr., D. Dai, A. Hernandez, and G. C. Fonarow, "Lipid Levels in Patients Hospitalized with Coronary Artery Disease: An Analysis of 136,905 Hospitalizations in Get with the Guidelines," *American Heart Journal* 157, no. 1 (January 2009): 111–117.

28.   US Food and Drug Administration, "Final Determination Regarding Partially Hydrogenated Oils (Removing Trans Fat)," May 18, 2018, https://www.fda.gov/food/food-additives-petitions/final -determination-regarding-partially-hydrogenated-oils -removing-trans-fat.

29.   G. L. King, *Reverse Your Diabetes in 12 Weeks: The Scientifically Proven Program to Avoid, Control, and Turn Around Your Diabetes* (New York: Workman, 2016).

30.   H. Kaplan, R. C. Thompson, B. C. Trumble, L. S. Wann, A. H. Allam, B. Beheim, B. Frohlich, et al., "Coronary Atherosclerosis in Indigenous South American Tsimane: A Cross-sectional Cohort Study," *Lancet* 389, no. 10080 (April 2017): 1730–1739.

31.   T. C. Campbell, *The China Study: The Most Comprehensive Study of Nutrition Ever Conducted and the Startling Implications for Diet, Weight Loss and Long-Term Health* (Dallas, TX: BenBella Books, 2006).

32.   C. Khambatta and R. Barbaro, *Mastering Diabetes: The Revolutionary Method to Reverse Insulin Resistance Permanently in Type 1, Type 1.5, Type 2, Prediabetes, and Gestational Diabetes* (New York: Avery, 2020).

33.   G. Taubes, *Good Calories, Bad Calories: Fats, Carbs, and the Controversial Science of Diet and Health* (New York: Anchor Books, 2008).

34. F. F. Samaha, N. Iqbal, P. Seshadri, K. L. Chicano, D. A. Daily, J. McGrory, T. Williams, et al., "A Low-Carbohydrate as Compared with a Low-Fat Diet in Severe Obesity," *New England Journal of Medicine* 348, no. 21 (May 2003): 2074–2081.

35. Another couple of examples are G. D. Foster, H. R. Wyatt, J. O. Hill, B. G. McGuckin, C. Brill, S. Mohammed, P. O. Szapary, et al., "A Randomized Trial of a Low-Carbohydrate Diet for Obesity," *New England Journal of Medicine* 348, no. 21 (June 2003): 2082–2090, and L. Stern, N. Iqbal, P. Seshadri, K. L. Chicano, D. A. Daily, J. McGrory, M. Williams, E. J. Gracely, and F. F. Samaha, "The Effects of Low-Carbohydrate versus Conventional Weight Loss Diets in Severely Obese Adults: One-Year Follow-Up of a Randomized Trial," *Annals of Internal Medicine* 140, no. 10 (May 2004): 778–785.

36. W. C. Willett, *Eat, Drink, and Be Healthy: The Harvard Medical School Guide to Healthy Eating* (New York: Simon and Schuster, 2001).

37. W. C. Hsu, K. H. K. Lau, M. Matsumoto, D. Moghazy, H. Keenan, and G. L. King, "Improvement of Insulin Sensitivity by Isoenergy High Carbohydrate Traditional Asian Diet: A Randomized Controlled Pilot Feasibility Study," *PLoS ONE* 9, no. 9 (September 2014): e106851, https://doi.org/10.1371/journal.pone.0106851.

38. K. Gunnars, "6 Things the World's Most Successful Diets Have in Common," *Healthline*, February 22, 2019, https://www.healthline.com/nutrition/6-things-successful-diets-have-in-common.

39. "Diabetic Exchange Diet," Drugs.com, February 3, 2020, https://www.drugs.com/cg/diabetic-exchange-diet.html.

CHAPTER 6

1. W. O. Atwater, *Foods: Nutritive Value and Cost* (Washington, DC: US Department of Agriculture, 1894), https://archive.org/details/CAT87201446.

2. C. B. Martin, K. A. Herrick, N. Sarafrazi, and C. L. Ogden, "Attempts to Lose Weight among Adults in the United States, 2013–2016," *NCHS Data Brief*, no. 313 (July 2018), https://www.cdc.gov/nchs/products/databriefs/db313.htm.

3.   R. K. Bernstein, *The Diabetes Diet: Dr. Bernstein's Low-Carbohydrate Solution* (New York: Little, Brown, 2005).

4.   G. L. King, *Reverse Your Diabetes in 12 Weeks: The Scientifically Proven Program to Avoid, Control, and Turn Around Your Diabetes* (New York: Workman, 2016).

5.   J. Bailor, *The Calorie Myth: How to Eat More, Exercise Less, Lose Weight, and Live Better* (New York: Harper Wave, 2014).

6.   Bernstein, *The Diabetes Diet.*

7.   US Department of Agriculture, "Nutrient Intakes from Food: Mean Amounts Consumed per Individual, by Gender and Age, in the United States, 2009–2010," in *What We Eat in America: NHANES 2009–2010* (Washington, DC: US Department of Agriculture, 2012), https://www.ars.usda.gov/Sp2userfiles/Place/12355000/Pdf/0910/Table_1_Nin_Gen_09.Pdf.

8.   J. W. Anderson, P. Baird, R. H. Davis Jr., S. Ferreri, M. Knudtson, A. Koraym, V. Waters, and C. L. Williams, "Health Benefits of Dietary Fiber," *Nutrition Reviews* 67, no. 4 (April 2009): 188–205.

9.   M. J. Clark and J. L. Slavin, "The Effect of Fiber on Satiety and Food Intake: A Systematic Review," *Journal of the American College of Nutrition* 32, no. 3 (2013): 200–211.

10.   E. Jovanovski, R. Khayyat, A. Zurbau, A. Komishon, N. Mazhar, J. L. Sievenpiper, S. B. Mejia, et al., "Should Viscous Fiber Supplements Be Considered in Diabetes Control? Results from a Systematic Review and Meta-analysis of Randomized Controlled Trials," *Diabetes Care* 42, no. 5 (May 2019): 755–766.

11.   *Mirakay v. Dakota Growers Pasta Co.*, Civil Action No. 13-cv-4429 (JAP) (D.N.J. Oct. 20, 2014).

12.   S. Schlender, "High-Fiber Foods and Blood Sugar—Quest Protein Bar Interview," *Me and My Diabetes*, March 3, 2012, http://www.meandmydiabetes.com/2012/03/03/high-fiber-foods-and-blood-sugar-quest-protein-bar-interview/.

13.   R. K. Bernstein, *The Diabetes Diet: Dr. Bernstein's Low-Carbohydrate Solution* (New York: Little, Brown, 2005).

14.   Ibid.

15. M. Pollan, *Food Rules: An Eater's Manual* (New York: Penguin Books, 2011).

CHAPTER 7

1. American Heart Association, "American Heart Association Recommendations for Physical Activity in Adults and Kids," April 18, 2018, https://www.heart.org/en/healthy-living/fitness/fitness-basics/aha-recs-for-physical-activity-in-adults.

2. S. R. Colberg, R. J. Sigal, J. E. Yardley, M. C. Riddell, D. W. Dunstan, P. C. Dempsey, E. S. Horton, K. Castorino, and D. F. Tate, "Physical Activity/Exercise and Diabetes: A Position Statement of the American Diabetes Association," *Diabetes Care* 39, no. 11 (November 2016): 2065–2079.

3. US Department of Health and Human Services, *Physical Activity Guidelines for Americans*, 2nd ed. (Washington, DC: US Department of Health and Human Services, 2018), https://health.gov/sites/default/files/2019-09/Physical_Activity_Guidelines_2nd_edition.pdf.

4. MyFitnessPal, "Calories Burned from Exercise," accessed June 19, 2020, https://www.myfitnesspal.com/exercise/lookup.

5. J. G. Thomas, D. S. Bond, S. Phelan, J. O. Hill, and R. R. Wing, "Weight-Loss Maintenance for 10 Years in the National Weight Control Registry," *American Journal of Preventive Medicine* 46, no. 1 (January 2014): 17–23.

6. J. A. Kanaley, S. R. Colberg, M. H. Corcoran, S. K. Malin, N. R. Rodriguez, C. J. Crespo, J. P. Kirwan, and J. R. Zierath, "Exercise/Physical Activity in Individuals with Type 2 Diabetes: A Consensus Statement from the American College of Sports Medicine," *Medicine and Science in Sports and Exercise* 54, no. 2 (February 2022): 353–368.

7. M. Zhao, S. P. Veeranki, S. Li, L. M. Steffen, and B. Xi, "Beneficial Associations of Low and Large Doses of Leisure-Time Physical Activity with All-Cause, Cardiovascular Disease and Cancer Mortality: A National Cohort Study of 88,140 U.S. Adults," *British Journal of Sports Medicine* 53, no. 22 (November 2019): 1405–1411.

8. P. F. Saint-Maurice, R. P. Troiano, D. R. Bassett Jr., B. I. Graubard, S. A. Carlson, E. J. Shiroma, J. E. Fulton, and C. E. Matthews, "Association of Daily Step Count and Step Intensity with Mortality among U.S. Adults," *JAMA* 323, no. 12 (2020): 1151–1160.

9. S. R. Colberg and American Diabetes Association, *Diabetes and Keeping Fit for Dummies* (Hoboken, NJ: Wiley, 2018).

10. S. Lu, "5 Keys to Putting the Fun in Fitness," *Diabetes Forecast*, May 2020.

11. G. Scheiner, "Sports and Exercise: The Ultimate Challenge in Blood Sugar Control," DiaTribe Learn, August 31, 2010, https://diatribe.org/sports-and-exercise-ultimate-challenge-blood-sugar-control.

12. American Diabetes Association, "Exercise and Type 1," accessed June 19, 2020, https://diabetes.org/fitness/get-and-stay-fit/exercise-and-type-1.

13. G. Vieira and J. Smith, *Pregnancy with Type 1 Diabetes: Your Month-to-Month Guide to Blood Sugar Management* (self-published, CreateSpace, 2017).

14. Intermountain Healthcare, "Food Adjustments for Exercise with Diabetes," 2016, https://intermountainhealthcare.org/ckr-ext/Dcmnt?ncid=520429251.

15. M. L. Erickson, N. T. Jenkins, and K. K. McCully, "Exercise after You Eat: Hitting the Postprandial Glucose Target," *Frontiers in Endocrinology (Lausanne)* 8 (September 2017): 228.

CHAPTER 8

1. J. R. White Jr., "A Brief History of the Development of Diabetes Medications," *Diabetes Spectrum* 27, no. 2 (May 2014): 82–86.

2. K. J. Quinn and N. H. Shah, "A Dataset Quantifying Polypharmacy in the United States," *Scientific Data* 4 (October 2017): 170167.

3. White, "A Brief History of the Development of Diabetes Medications."

4. C. L. Maikawa, A. A. A. Smith, L. Zou, G. A. Roth, E. C. Gale, L. M. Stapleton, S. W. Baker, et al., "A Co-formulation of Supramolecularly Stabilized Insulin and Pramlintide Enhances Mealtime Glucagon Suppression in Diabetic Pigs," *Nature Biomedical Engineering* 4 (May 2020): 507–517.

5. Centers for Disease Control and Prevention, *National Diabetes Statistics Report, 2020: Estimates of Diabetes and Its Burden in the United States* (Atlanta, GA: Centers for Disease Control and Prevention, 2020).

6. A. K. Lee, B. Warren, C. J. Lee, J. W. McEvoy, K. Matsushita, E. S. Huang, A. R. Sharrett, J. Coresh, and E. Selvin, "The Association of Severe Hypoglycemia with Incident Cardiovascular Events and Mortality in Adults with Type 2 Diabetes," *Diabetes Care* 41, no. 1 (January 2018): 104–111.

7. P. E. Cryer, "Severe Hypoglycemia Predicts Mortality in Diabetes," *Diabetes Care* 35, no. 9 (September 2012): 1814–1816.

8. R. K. Bernstein, *Dr. Bernstein's Diabetes Solution: The Complete Guide to Achieving Normal Blood Sugars*, 4th ed. (New York: Little, Brown Spark, 2011).

9. L. Heinemann, C. Weyer, M. Rauhaus, S. Heinrichs, and T. Heise, "Variability of the Metabolic Effect of Soluble Insulin and the Rapid-Acting Insulin Analog Insulin Aspart," *Diabetes Care* 21, no. 11 (November 1998): 1910–1914.

10. C. Zehrer, R. Hansen, and John Bantle, "Reducing Blood Glucose Variability by Use of Abdominal Insulin Injection Sites," *Diabetes Educator* 16, no. 6 (November–December 1990): 474–477.

11. D. J. Kumbhani, "Dapagliflozin and Prevention of Adverse Outcomes in Chronic Kidney Disease—DAPA-CKD," American College of Cardiology, August 23, 2021, https://www.acc.org/latest-in-cardiology/clinical-trials/2020/08/28/17/07/dapa-ckd.

12. US Food and Drug Administration, "FDA Drug Safety Communication: FDA Strengthens Kidney Warnings for Diabetes Medicines Canagliflozin (Invokana, Invokamet) and Dapagliflozin (Farxiga, Xigduo XR)," June 14, 2016, https://www.fda.gov/drugs/drug-safety-and-availability/fda-drug-safety-communication-fda-strengthens-kidney-warnings-diabetes-medicines-canagliflozin.

13. Diabetes Teaching Center, "Table of Medications," *Diabetes Education Online*, accessed June 19, 2020, https://dtc.ucsf.edu/types-of-diabetes/ type2/treatment-of-type-2-diabetes/medications-and-therapies/ type-2-non-insulin-therapies/table-of-medications/.

14. J. P. Cunha, "Metformin," RxList, September 21, 2021, https://www .rxlist.com/consumer_metformin/drugs-condition.htm.

15. See the Drugs.com "Drug Interactions Checker," at https://www .drugs.com/drug_interactions.html.

16. M. Monami, C. Nardini, and E. Mannucci, "Efficacy and Safety of Sodium Glucose Co-Transport-2 Inhibitors in Type 2 Diabetes: A Meta-analysis of Randomized Clinical Trials," *Diabetes, Obesity and Metabolism* 16, no. 5 (May 2014): 457–466.

17. J. Rosenstock, S. Perl, E. K. Johnsson, and S. Jacob, "Triple vs. Dual Therapy with Low-Dose Dapagliflozin Plus Saxagliptin vs. Each Monocomponent Added to Metformin in Uncontrolled Type 2 Diabetes," Supplement 1, *Diabetes* 67 (July 2018): 1149-P.

18. R. Schroeder, T. D. Harrison, and S. L. McGraw, "Treatment of Adult Obesity with Bariatric Surgery," *American Family Physician*, 93, no. 1 (2018): 31–37.

19. American Diabetes Association, "Economic Costs of Diabetes in the U.S. in 2017," *Diabetes Care* 41, no. 5 (May 2018): 917–928, https:// doi.org/10.2337/dci18-0007.

20. Right Care Alliance, "High Insulin Costs Are Killing Americans," accessed June 19, 2020, https://rightcarealliance.org/actions/insulin/.

21. D. K. Roberts, "The Deadly Costs of Insulin," *American Journal of Managed Care*, June 10, 2019, https://www.ajmc.com/view/ the-deadly-costs-of-insulin.

22. K. Mui, "The GoodRx List Price Index Reveals the Rising Cost of All Diabetes Treatments—Not Just Insulin," GoodRx, April 10, 2019, https://www.goodrx.com/blog/goodrx-list-price-index-rising-cost-of -diabetes-treatments/.

23. GoodRx, "Dapagliflozin," accessed June 19, 2020, https://www.goodrx .com/dapagliflozin.

24. GoodRx, "Wegovy," accessed July 1, 2021, https://www.goodrx.com/ wegovy.

25. K. Lipska, "Break Up the Insulin Racket," *New York Times*, February 20, 2016, https://www.nytimes.com/2016/02/21/opinion/sunday/break-up-the-insulin-racket.html.

26. W. T. Cefalu, D. E. Dawes, G. Gavlak, D. Goldman, W. H. Herman, K. Van Nuys, A. C. Powers, S. I. Taylor, and A. L. Yatvin, "Insulin Access and Affordability Working Group: Conclusions and Recommendations," *Diabetes Care* 41, no. 6 (June 2018): 1299–1311.

27. P. Callaghan, "'A Great Day': Minnesota Legislature Finally Passes Emergency Insulin Bill," *Minnpost*, April 15, 2020, https://www.minnpost.com/state-government/2020/04/a-great-day-minnesota-legislature-finally-passes-emergency-insulin-bill/.

28. National Association of Boards of Pharmacy, "Internet Drug Outlet Identification Program: Progress Report for State and Federal Regulators, August 2017," 2017, https://nabp.pharmacy/wp-content/uploads/2016/08/Internet-Drug-Outlet-Report-August-2017.pdf.

29. GoodRx, "Metformin," accessed June 19, 2020, https://www.goodrx.com/metformin.

30. Mui, "The GoodRx List Price Index."

31. S. W. Ponder and K. L. McMahon, *Sugar Surfing: How to Manage Type 1 Diabetes in a Modern World* (Sausalito, CA: Mediself Press, 2015).

CHAPTER 9

1. R. Greenberg, "Dexcom Clarity App's Malfunction," *Diabetes Stories*, March 23, 2022, https://diabetesstories.com/2022/03/23/dexcoms-clarity-apps-mistake/.

2. R. K. Bernstein, "Children with Diabetes—Q&A," *Dr. Bernstein's Diabetes Solution*, March 1998, http://www.diabetes-book.com/children-diabetes-qa/.

INDEX

H

I

Index

medication therapy management, 162–163, 165. *See also* drugs for diabetes management

meglitinides, 132

mental part of diabetes care

in current hierarchy of care, 22, 27–29

desserts and fast food, 46–47

fallacy of normalcy, 47–50

futility of going on a diet, 59–66

Ginger Vieira on, 71–76

homeostasis and, 54–56

in ideal hierarchy of care, 30

language of diabetes, 50–52

motivation, 40–42

overview of, 40

questions for care providers, 52, 76–77

sugar consumption and, 42–46

twelve-step perspective, 66–71

weight loss as by-product of healthy living, 56–59

metabolic syndrome

and cardiovascular disease, 90

double diabetics, 11

and high-carb, high-fat diet, 85

and high-carb, low-fat diet, 93

and low-carb diets, 93

questions for care providers, 76

type 2 diabetes, 7–8

metformin, 9, 149, 150

Metropolitan Life Insurance, 105

Mission Carb Balance tortillas, 113

money, saving, 152–156

motivation, 40–42, 128–129

Muccioli, Maria, 100

MyPlate (USDA), 25

N

Nathan, David, 43

National Institutes of Health (NIH) funding, 14

National Weight Control Registry (NWCR), 63–65

net carbs, 60–61, 110–113

NMR LipoProfile panel, 99

normal eating. *See also* nutrition

fallacy of normalcy, 47–50

as impossible with diabetes, 41–42

nutrition. *See also* low-carb eating

blood sugar average and time in range, 81–84

building diet, 114–116

calories and, 104–106, 107–109

care provider training in, 22

consulting care provider when changing, 55

in current hierarchy of care, 21, 22, 24–26

desserts, 45, 46–47, 48

and devices for diabetes management, 156–157

dietary fat as healthy, 89–91

dietary fiber and, 109–113

dynamic blood sugar management, 157–161, 168–171

and exercise, 126, 136

experimenting with approaches to, 74–75

fallacy of normalcy, 47–50

fast food, 45, 46–47, 85

finding healthy macronutrient balance, 84–95

focusing on, over drugs, 147–156

futility of going on a diet, 59–66

goals of diabetic, 80

high-carb, high-fat diet, 84–85, 119

high-carb, low-fat diet, 91–92, 93–97, 108, 110, 114

red meat, 94

refined carbs, 96–98. *See also* carbohydrates; sugar

ReliOn brand insulin products, 153

resilience, 71–75

resistance training, 133–134

routine, importance of daily, 170

rules for healthy eating, 95–98. *See also* nutrition

Runyan, Keith, 88

rural Asian diet (RAD), 91–92, 108

S

SAD (standard American diet), 84, 119

safety in exercise, 130–133

saturated fat, 89–90, 97

saving money by using less medication, 152–156

scheduling exercise for health, 136–138

self-monitoring, 64, 65

Semglee, 153

side effects, 147–149, 163

Smith, Alec, 152

spiritual component of twelve-step philosophy, 68

standard American diet (SAD), 84, 119

Stanislaw, Jody, 116–122

The Starch Solution (McDougall), 79

Stefansson, Vilhjalmur, 87

sugar. *See also* blood sugar; carbohydrates
  addictiveness of, 44–45
  desserts, 45, 46–47, 48
  fallacy of normalcy, 47–50
  fast food, 45, 46–47, 85
  Jody Stanislaw on, 120–121
  myth related to eating, 42–46
  rules for healthy eating, 96–98

sugar alcohols, 111, 113

"Sugar Is Not a Treat" (Stanislaw), 122

Sugar Surfing, 157–158

Sugar Surfing (Ponder and McMahon), 161

sulfonylureas, 131–132

supplementation, fiber, 110

supply chain, diabetes medication, 153–154

support groups, 27–28

support in twelve-step perspective, 68

sushi, 49

T

Taking Control of Your Diabetes (TCOYD) conferences, 18–19, 24–25, 46–47, 50

Taubes, Gary, 55

teenagers with diabetes, 171

thriving with diabetes, 73–75

time in range, 57, 82, 169

tirzepatide, 151

T1D. *See* diabetes management; type 1 diabetes

T1D Crew, 122

training for patients with diabetes, 27

trans fats, 89–91, 97

Tsimané people, 92

T2D. *See* diabetes management; type 2 diabetes

twelve-step perspective in managing diabetes, 29, 66–71, 169. *See also* devices for diabetes management; diet; drugs for diabetes management; exercise; mental part of diabetes care

type 1 diabetes (T1D). *See also* diabetes management
  complexity of, 12
  Jody Stanislaw's work related to, 121–122
  overview of, 10–11

ABOUT THE AUTHOR

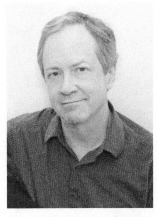

CHAD T. LEWIS spent a career in higher education, at different times as a counselor, dean, and professor. Chad earned two graduate degrees, one in business and the other in education. He coauthored business courseware and management textbooks for major publishers (McGraw-Hill, Harcourt-Brace, and Allyn and Bacon) and published research in peer-reviewed journals in the human resources, management, and education fields. He became a Joslin Medalist in 2018, having survived type 1 diabetes for more than fifty years. Chad lives on Camano Island in Washington State with his wife, Patty.

Made in the USA
Las Vegas, NV
20 November 2022